AIR CRASHES
AND
MIRACLE LANDINGS
PART 2
Large Print Edition

Air Crashes and Miracle Landings is a great resource for every pilot who wants a clear summary of the whats, hows, and whys behind the key aviation accidents.

This book should be part of Human Factors and Crew Resource Management training.

Richard de Crespigny
Captain of QF32

AIR CRASHES
AND
MIRACLE LANDINGS
PART 2
Large Print Edition

By
Christopher Bartlett

ISBN 978-0-9560723-8-2

© January 2019

OpenHatch Books,
Gillingham, Dorset, UK
mail@openhatchbooks.com
https://chrisbart.com

Cover
by
Lysa Bartlett

PREFACE

The original Air *Crashes and Miracle Landings*, with all 85 key incidents, remains the ideal Quick Reference Handbook (QRH) for professionals or even fans of the *Air Accident Investigations/MAYDAY* TV series. Having the whole book in one volume facilitates searches, especially on the Kindle.

On the other hand, readers going right through the printed book studying the whys and hows in detail will perhaps prefer this *large-print* edition. A good present for those who remember the headlines at the time and always wondered what really happened.

Chapters 1-7 of the original book are in Part 1, and Chapters 8-18 in Part 2. Updates and the glossary (which we had to omit for lack of space) are in Part 3 for which there is also a Kindle version.

For all those who died
and all those who survived.

Lessons were learned
for the benefit
of us all.

Table of Contents

FIGURES

Diagrams and images are included only where essential for explanation, since so many, even in color, can be easily found on the Internet.

On the Kindle, images may appear small but can usually be expanded to show finer detail.

x

Chapter 8
PILOT ISSUES

Uptight BEA Trident Captain's Heart Attack (Staines, 1972)

Fear-instilling captain and diffident rookie first officer

> Lack of a cockpit voice recording made it impossible to determine who did what in the following incident. Graffiti critical of the captain who had been involved in a furious argument in the crew room before departure was found in the cockpit.
>
> British European Airways Flight 548, June 18, 1972

The British European Airways trijet Trident had taken off for Brussels from London's Heathrow airport in cloudy and somewhat turbulent weather. Only 114 seconds into its flight, with the aircraft traveling at 162 knots at about 1,500 feet, someone moved the lever controlling the leading-edge droops, causing them to retract.

Droops, as their name implies, are like upper lips on the front (leading edges) of the wings that can be made to droop forward and downward to change the configuration of the wing and enable the aircraft to fly at low airspeeds. Their function is like that of the much better-known slats.

For the aircraft to be able to fly without the droops deployed the airspeed would have had to be at least 15 to 20 knots higher than the 162 knots at which they were flying. In fact, to allow a safety margin, the pilots would only retract the droops once the airspeed had reached

225 knots, and never when the aircraft was in a turn which it was, as an aircraft is more vulnerable in a turn, especially if the turn involves turning away from a strong headwind since the drop in airspeed can be dramatic. Every Trident pilot would have had this minimum droop retraction speed drummed into him or her and could hardly forget it, as it was in addition indicated next to the droop lever.

Even so, retracting the droops by mistake need not prove immediately fatal, as even in those days airliners had good systems to warn pilots of an imminent stall. Sensors on the wings would detect development of abnormal airflow over the leading edge, and a stick shaker system would shake the control columns to warn the pilots. According to the flight data recorder (FDR), on that BEA flight the stick shaker operated less than two seconds after retraction of the droops.

Furthermore, aircraft like the Trident, with the engines at the rear and high tails (high horizontal stabilizers), are equipped with a stick pusher system that pushes the nose down in a stall. This is to compensate for the fact that aircraft with engines at the rear and high tails go nose-up rather than nose-down in a stall, thus making the stall worse and often irrecoverable if anywhere near the ground.

Apart from in cases of extreme wind shear, an aircraft's airspeed changes progressively, so that in normal circumstances the stick shaker warning (that the airspeed is falling to such an extent that a stall is imminent) occurs well before the last resort stick push.

However, as this was a "change-of-configuration stall"—that is, not due to a progressive drop in airspeed but due to a change in the shape of the wing—these events took place so quickly that the stick shake warning and stick push must have seemed to have occurred almost simultaneously.

The virtual concurrence of these two events may have confused the pilots, for when the stick push mechanism duly caused the nose to pitch downward, and so much so that the aircraft gained almost sufficient speed to recover, someone fought against the stick pusher and pulled the nose up. Once more the stick pusher operated to push the nose down, only for someone again to use considerable force to resist it, before finally disabling it. As at no point was there any attempt made to increase engine power, one must conclude that whoever was at the controls was unaware of the true situation.

With the nose yanked up again without redeployment of the droops and no application of additional power, the Trident did what the stick pusher was trying to prevent—it went into a deep, unrecoverable tail-down stall.

Below them a thirteen-year-old boy walking with his younger brother along a footpath saw the Trident with its wings level drop out of the cloud above with the tail, weighed down by its three heavy engines, striking the ground first and breaking off. The rest of the aircraft then belly flopped onto the field with the sound of crumpling and tearing metal as the fuselage and wings separated into various pieces. Despite the large amount of fuel carried at takeoff spilling onto the ground, there was no fire—no doubt because of the lack of forward speed.

With air traffic controllers not even having noticed the aircraft's disappearance, the boy ran to a house some four hundred yards away for help. The occupant rushed to the scene, but her skills as a hospital emergency room nurse were of little avail, as only one person showed any sign of life, and that sole survivor later died in hospital, making the total death toll 118. The official report into the crash praised her highly.

There have been survivors in crashes, even with intense fires, where the wreckage must have looked even worse. However, with the wings providing no lift at all and the forward speed dissipated by the drag produced by the nose-up/tail-down attitude, the Trident had belly flopped almost straight down, with virtually nothing between the occupants and the ground to cushion the shock. Had the aircraft belly flopped on the nearby trees, they might have absorbed enough of the shock to enable some to survive.

1. Someone had retracted the droops before the aircraft had reached sufficient airspeed to stay in the air without them and, contrary to company regulations, when the aircraft was in a banked turn and more vulnerable.
2. The built-in stall warnings (stick shaker) were ignored, and the automatic recovery (stick pusher) resisted several times before being disabled.
3. Inexplicably, at almost every stage of the short flight, prior to and including the fatal retraction of

the droops, the airspeed had been lower than it should have been, and this unusually low airspeed had made the retraction of the droops especially lethal.

4.   The captain, who was handling the aircraft, had had a heart attack, and medical experts concluded from the color of the blood in his heart that he was probably dead before the aircraft hit the ground.

The Investigation

The investigators had to resort almost entirely to supposition, as the aircraft did not have a cockpit voice recorder (CVR), even though CVRs had been made mandatory for US-registered airliners much earlier in 1965. (Opposition from the UK pilots' unions had thwarted their introduction in the UK.)

It was impossible to know who did what and why. From terse communications with ATC, it was evident that the captain had been handling the aircraft, but it was not clear who had moved the droop lever.

The initial investigation was followed by a public inquiry, with lawyers arguing for days without producing anything of significance that was not apparent from the original investigation. What were apparent, as in so many crashes, were the human personality factors that experience has shown increase the likelihood of a disaster.

On the flight deck there were four pilots:

1.   Captain Key, an uptight captain, who supported the company in the ongoing industrial dispute.

2. Twenty-two-year-old Second Officer Keighley. He had only very few hours' line experience on the Trident. He was in the first officer's seat next to the captain.
3. Twenty-four-year-old Second Officer Ticehurst, who was in the monitoring seat.
4. A Captain Collins in the jump seat behind Captain Key. This second captain was deadheading with his own crew to Brussels. Although a freighter captain on another aircraft type, he too was qualified to fly Tridents.

Though technically qualified, Keighley was thought by instructors, both before and after joining the airline, to lack initiative and to be rather diffident. While they thought he would eventually make a good pilot, his relatively young age, unassertive character, and inexperience meant he would have trouble coping with a captain known to be uptight

Industrial action at the airline meant that some junior pilots had not had the extra training required to permit them to legally occupy the third seat (behind the captain and first officer). He or she would be monitoring the flying pilot's actions and performing certain technical functions that used to be done by a flight engineer and necessitated the extra paper qualifications. This quirk in the regulations in turn meant that the least qualified pilot was likely to be at the controls next to the captain.

Furthermore, prior to the flight, Captain Key had been involved in a violent argument in the crew room with another pilot about the strike, and Keighley had witnessed the captain's violent outburst of temper. In addition, it was said that the considerable air turbulence must have raised Keighley's certainly already high stress level.

The investigators thought the presence of Captain Collins in the jump seat might have distracted the junior pilots. The official report notes that when Captain Collins was found in the debris, he was still holding an air freshener can in his hand. These air fresheners were standard issue for freighter captains, but one wonders what he was doing with it so early in the flight. Was Captain Key sweating so profusely that use of the air freshener was deemed necessary? An awful possibility that no one hitherto has suggested is that Captain Collins was standing up with his air freshener, and this had been a further distraction. He might even have fallen forward when the initial stick push occurred, blocking the view of Ticehurst.

In his book *Disaster in the Air*, Jan Bartelski, who has worked in senior positions for the International Airline Pilots' Association, says an official accident report should not publicize details such as being found dead grasping an air freshener. However, in the author's opinion it does seem very relevant in that many people have said that Captain Collins's body being found without earphones, slumped away from his seat, might mean he was trying to get to the droop lever to reset the droops. Would he have done this with the air freshener can in his hand?

Jan Bartelski does postulate that an erroneous airspeed reading on the captain's side might have led him to retract the droops because he thought they were going too fast rather than too slow. This would account for the consistently low airspeeds at the various stages of the short flight, which no one can explain, apart from suggesting this resulted from the captain being in pain.

Possible Contributory Causes
1. The airline's training.
2. Reports of similar incidents being overlooked because of bureaucratic muddle, staff absence (holidays), and bad luck.

Outstanding Questions
1. Why was the aircraft flying more slowly than it should have been at various stages of the climb-out?
2. Why was the droop lever moved?
3. In addition, why, even if the captain was incapacitated, didn't the other two pilots, and especially the monitoring pilot, realize what was happening?

As a result, the British government belatedly made the installation of cockpit voice recorders mandatory, as in the US.

Korean Air Cargo Flight Banks Too Far (Stanstead, 1999)

Aware of danger copilot did not dare question ex-colonel

> This crash had something in common with the disaster just described: a crusty senior captain and junior inexperienced copilot.
>
> Korean Air Cargo Flight 8509, December 22, 1999

At the time of this incident, Korean Airlines had a culture quite the opposite of that practiced through cockpit resource management (CRM) in Western airlines. Firstly, Korean culture meant that younger people obeyed their elders even when not agreeing. Secondly, most pilots were ex-military, and in the military disobeying orders was not tolerated.

Korean Air Cargo Flight 8509 took off from London's Stanstead Airport in the early evening of December 22, 1999. The captain was a former colonel in the Korean Air Force with 13,490 flying hours, of which 8,495 were on the Boeing 747. As was the custom, senior officers such as he were catapulted to the rank of captain and had little understanding of flying as part of a team.

His copilot had only 195 flight hours on the 747 out of a total of 1,406. The flight engineer, however, was very experienced. A Korean technician was also on board.

On the leg to Stanstead, with different pilots, a fault with one of the aircraft's inertial guidance systems disabled the attitude indicator on the captain's side. This, an artificial horizon, indicates whether the nose is pointing up or down and whether the aircraft is banking to the left or right. As it was daylight, there was the natural horizon outside to help the pilots. Unfortunately, repairs at Stanstead did not correct the problem.

The aircraft lifted off normally from the Stanstead runway, but after 16.7 seconds, the comparator warned of the attitude indicator discrepancy for the first time. The first officer called for a heading of 158 degrees, with the comparator warning having sounded again. The captain turned the control wheel through 30 degrees to the left twenty-nine seconds after takeoff, although the flight engineer had called out "Bank is not working," and the roll attitude was already 46.5 degrees. The captain moved the control wheel back to neutral as the aircraft approached their intended heading but made no further adjustment, presumably because his attitude indicator showed no bank.

Fifty seconds after takeoff, the captain, oblivious to the fact that their derived roll to the left was 80.6 degrees, requested radar vectors.

Data ended five seconds later with them having dropped to 1,042 feet, and at an airspeed of 262 knots, a downward pitch of 35.5 degrees, and a derived roll attitude of 72.3 to the left. The aircraft crashed, killing all four on board. Though his life was at risk, the copilot had not dared question his superior's actions.

Aftermath

Korean Air modified its piloting culture at the instigation of the incensed South Korean president and, with the help of Delta, became one of the safest airlines.

Overcontrolling Copilot Swishes off Airbus Tail (NYC, 2001)

Why him? Two months after 9/11

> Though wake turbulence was a key factor in this incident, it has been included in this chapter, as it was a propensity of the first officer, perhaps accentuated by his training, that was most likely the cause.
>
> American Airlines Flight 587, November 12, 2001

The sixteen-thousand-foot runway at Denver International Airport in Colorado is the longest commercial runway in North America. It owes this distinction to the city literally being a mile high and thus needing an exceptionally long runway to cope with heavily laden aircraft that accelerate less quickly at the lower atmospheric pressures found at high altitudes.

The previous record holder, the slightly shorter 14,572-foot (4,441-meter) Runway 31L at New York's JFK airport, probably still holds the record for the best takeoff prospects, as it is at sea level, as well as being exceptionally long.

A drawback of New York's 31L is that the city lies straight ahead, albeit in the distance. To avoid areas that are sensitive for noise and other reasons, including terrorist action, aircraft taking off in that northwesterly (310-degree) direction usually have to make a sharp left turn shortly after takeoff so as to avoid the city and fly mostly over water. Air traffic controllers would often warn of the danger of wake turbulence, especially from heavily laden jumbo jets such as the Boeing 747.

Wake turbulence consists of vicious vortices of swirling air produced at the wingtips, where the air squished under the wings meets the lower-pressure, relatively fast-moving air above them. These hang behind the aircraft, and, spinning like tops, gradually descend, until their energy either dissipates or they are broken up by other turbulence. In fact, turbulent or stormy weather conditions help protect following aircraft from wake turbulence, as the turbulence breaks up the spirals. It is in calm conditions that wake turbulence is the most treacherous.

On November 12, 2001, almost two months to the day after 9/11, with the images of the two hijacked aircraft slamming into the World Trade Center's twin towers still vivid in people's minds, Japan Airlines Flight JL47 to Tokyo took off from runway 31L at JFK. It was just after 9:00 a.m. The shorter, parallel runway, 31R, on the other side of the terminal buildings was being used for incoming aircraft, including the soon expected British Airways supersonic Concorde Flight 1 from London.

That day, aircraft taking off on JFK's 31L were encountering a light headwind of just nine knots.

JL47 acknowledged the takeoff clearance from the tower but waited perhaps fifteen seconds longer than usual before beginning its roll. In addition, with the large amount of fuel required for the thirteen-hour-plus flight to Tokyo, it would have climbed out more slowly than most other 747s just hopping across the pond to Europe.

The tower had already warned a police helicopter to exercise caution about wake turbulence from several heavy jet departures over a suburb to the left of the runway extension[1] called Canarsie.

Once well into the air, the Japan Airlines pilots would retract the flaps and commence a high-power climb. It is precisely when climbing under high power with a clean configuration—that is, no flaps or slats sticking out—that a large aircraft, such as the 747, produces the most wake turbulence.

The next aircraft in line to take off was American Airlines Flight 587, an Airbus A300 bound for the Dominican Republic with 260 people on board, a flight expected to take some four hours but which in fact was to last only 104 seconds from liftoff. First Officer Sten Molin was the pilot flying (PF), with Captain Edward States in command. The tower had warned the A300 of the danger of wake turbulence, but this was routine in the circumstances. In fact, many considered it a phrase used to cover the controllers' backs, with the effect being somewhat like someone crying wolf too often. Nevertheless, Molin was obviously concerned, for he said to the captain:

You happy with that distance?

The captain replied:

Aah, he's . . . We'll be all right once we get rollin'. He's supposed to be five miles by the time we get airborne. That's the idea.

First officer:

So you're happy . . . Lights?

Captain:

Yeah, lights are on.

Preparations for takeoff continued.

First officer:

Takeoff checks complete. I'm on the roll. Thank you, sir.

The aircraft began its roll and reached the takeoff decision speed, V_1.

Captain:

V_1!

The aircraft then reached rotation speed, V_R.

Captain:

V_R!

Captain:

Rotate!

The captain confirmed they had reached the safe takeoff (climb) speed, V_2, and then V_2 +10 knots, giving them an extra safety margin.

First officer:

Positive rate. Gear up, please.

With the aircraft five hundred feet off the ground, the aircraft was banking left as the control tower ordered the crew to turn left and fly the bridge climb, like JL47 ahead of them. However, they had commenced their left turn earlier than JL47, with the result that they were cutting the corner downwind of the Japan Airlines craft rather than following in its precise tracks.

Also, in taking off with what seemed to the captain to be a just about acceptable gap between them and the Japan Airlines 747 ahead, he had not taken into account that they would be climbing much more quickly than the heavily fuel-laden Japan-bound jumbo.

The control tower signed off, telling the A300 to contact New York Departure (Control). They duly informed departure they were at thirteen hundred feet and climbing to five thousand. Departure confirmed they had them on their radar and said:

Climb. Maintain one three thousand.

They acknowledged this. The A300 passed through fifteen hundred feet at roughly 220 knots, and the bank eased as it completed its turn to the left. The Japan Airlines 747 was ahead of them but upwind and farther out on the curve and somewhat higher, but not so much higher, due to its load of fuel.

As Captain States and First Officer Molin passed through 1,769 feet at 239 knots, departure called, telling them to turn left again.

587 heavy, turn left . . .

The cockpit area microphone (CAM) picked up a squeak and a rattle.

Captain:

Little wake turbulence, huh?

[The wake turbulence from one of the JAL 747's wingtips.]

First officer:

Yeah!

The aircraft was in a steep but not excessive bank as it continued to make the second left turn as ordered. Fourteen seconds later, and traveling at 238 knots, it encountered the wake turbulence from the JAL 747's other wingtip.

In a strained voice, Molin asked for maximum power, and the following exchange took place between the two pilots, with Captain States speaking first:

You all right?

Yeah, I'm fine.

Hang on to it. Hang on to it.

This time the buffeting seemed more serious, and the flight data recorder (FDR) shows First Officer Molin continuously making rapid full-sweep, to-and-fro rudder inputs *in addition* to the aileron inputs that were normal for such a situation. In fact, the rudder is not used very much in general flying apart from compensating for a crosswind on landing with the aircraft traveling relatively slowly.

The cockpit area microphone (CAM) recorded the sound of a thump.

CAM:

[Loud thump.]

CAM:

[Loud bang.]

Molin:

[Human grunt?]

CAM:

[Roaring noise starts and becomes louder.]

Molin:

Holy s***!

There followed warning chimes, which were probably first ECAM chimes and then stall warning chimes.

[Roaring noise decreases and ceases.]

Molin:

What the hell are we into? . . . We're stuck in it.

[Possibly more chimes, lasting some four seconds overall.]

Captain:

Get out of it! Get out of it!

[End of recording.]

Loss of Tailfin and Crash

When Captain States was saying "Get out of it!" neither he nor Molin knew the vertical tail fin had broken off some fourteen seconds earlier and was falling into Jamaica Bay below.

The aircraft, minus its vertical stabilizer (tail fin), continued a little farther and crashed onto a narrow band of land separating Jamaica Bay from the Atlantic Ocean, which is part of Queens. None of the 260 people on board the Airbus 300 survived. The death toll on the ground could have been considerable as it was a residential neighborhood but was limited to five persons since most pieces hit unoccupied property or open spaces.

The big question was why Molin had swished the rudder back and forth in such a manner. The investigators had some difficulty determining just how extreme Molin's movements had been, because of the four-second sampling rate—that is, the frequency with which the FDR measures the angle of the rudder.

In that time it would have been possible for Molin to move the rudder back and forth without it showing up.

Another problem was that the readings, as are many others on FDRs, are filtered to avoid confusing spikes. This averaging would not matter when dealing with a rudder used in virtually one position, as would usually be the case, but obscured the magnitude of the extremes that investigators so much wanted to know in the present situation.

One major line of inquiry was obviously to find out whether the tail fin had some inherent weakness, either due to poor design or previous overstressing that had left undetected cracks. Since it was made of composites rather than the traditional metal, there was much talk that composite tail fins were inherently dangerous, partly because, unlike metal tail fins, cracks are so difficult to detect. Some American Airlines pilots even talked of boycotting the Airbus A300.

In the end, and after exhaustive examinations and tests, the investigators concluded the accident had not resulted from an inherent weakness but from Molin's aggressive use of the rudder, and in particular his rapidly moving it back and forth.[2]

The next question posed was why Molin had done this. Should the manufacturer have warned that doing so was dangerous? As large sums of money and prestige were at stake, there then ensued a battle between Airbus and American Airlines.

Investigators investigated Molin's personal life so extensively that his father, also a pilot, complained. Inquiries almost got to the point of ascertaining how Molin performed in bed. He was said to be a little immature socially, and his deferential manner in his exchanges with Captain States do hint at this. However, investigators found nothing dramatic. On the other hand, American Airlines argued Airbus knew of the dangers and had done too little to warn pilots.

Airbus maintained that the airline had trained Molin to use the rudder in recovery situations, and being nervous about wake turbulence even before takeoff, he expected it and overreacted when it occurred. Following this line of thought, one could say the first encounter keyed him up so that he was more aggressive the second time.

Some experts said that as he reacted mildly the first time, the turbulence the second time might have been rather different and produced the yawing movement to which he reacted instinctively by using the rudder.

Perverse though it might seem, had First Officer Molin been captain rather than first officer, the subsequent joust with wake turbulence might have never taken place. When Molin politely asked the captain just before takeoff whether he was happy with the distance between them and the JAL aircraft ahead, he was evidently thinking it would be better to wait perhaps thirty seconds more.

This expression of serious doubt to seniors in the form of a question brings to mind the worst-ever aircraft disaster, at Tenerife, where the flight engineer used the words "Did he not clear the runway then?"

Had Molin been less polite and said forcefully "I think we should wait a moment," the captain of Flight 587 might have done just that and not tried to justify himself.

Admittedly, the KLM flight engineer at Tenerife would have had to be very assertive to halt that fatal takeoff roll.

Conversely, had Captain States been flying the aircraft, his laid-back attitude would probably have meant he would have let the aircraft have its head and not have used the rudder so disastrously, if at all. However, his telling Molin "Hang on to it. Hang on to it!" might have made Molin even more determined to keep the aircraft on a leash, though "hang on" was not literally telling him to swish the rudder, but it could have been interpreted as that.

With hindsight, one can also see that had Flight 587 followed the track of the Japan Airlines 747 more closely instead of cutting the corner, as ordered by ATC, it would have missed the turbulence altogether, as it would have been blown downwind. In a sense, the required separation was not maintained once the corner was cut. Of course, the premature turn over water would subject built-up areas to less noise.

An article on a now-terminated website called **mywiseowl** half seriously said, "The primary purpose of flight data recorders (FDRs) is to reduce the manufacturer's liability by correctly assigning blame to the failing assemblies or persons, with the famous secondary purpose being to prevent future accidents."

Had FDR evidence not been available in this accident, would anyone have thought the first officer would have made those rudder movements? Thus, the FDR did indeed help save the day for the manufacturer.

NTSB's Final Report

The airline put considerable pressure on the investigators, making new points until they were told not to make new representations unless based on new facts. Whether or not this pressure was a factor in the change made to the order in which the contributory factors were listed, it is notable that board member Carol J. Carmody, with the concurrence of board member Richard F. Healing, added a dissenting statement to the report.

While they agreed with its conclusions as regards probable cause, namely the excessive use of the rudder by the first officer, they objected to the fact that the vice-chairman had changed the order in which the contributory causes were listed from that in the original draft. This gave the impression that more weight should be given to the characteristics of the A300 rudder system[3] than to the nature of the airline's Advanced Aircraft Maneuvering Program (AAMP).[4]

They pointed out that Molin had not been known to use the rudder abnormally before partaking in the program, and when questioned by a captain about excessive use of the rudder in another incident after taking part in the program, Molin had insisted the AAMP directed him to use the rudder in that manner. Carmody went on to say, "To elevate the characteristics of the A300-600 rudder system in the hierarchy of contributing factors ignores the fact that this system had not been an issue in sixteen million hours of testing and operator experience—until the AAMP-trained pilot flew it."

This puts Molin in a rather different light. Known as a hands-on pilot, with some saying his flying was as smooth as silk, maybe his only propensity or quirk was to follow things too much to the letter.

In 2012, and in the light of other cases where the A300 tail assembly had been subjected to excessive stress but not enough to cause it to break off, the NTSB said the A300 should have greater built-in protection against such events, which suggests they no longer think another pilot doing what Molin did is inconceivable. Though the initial report was not revised, it does suggest, as some investigators felt, Airbus bore some responsibility, though the airline's Advanced Aircraft Maneuvering Program (AAMP), involving application of significant rudder inputs, was surely a factor.

Interestingly, the latest advice to pilots, admittedly often destined for smaller craft, is to do absolutely nothing on encountering wake turbulence. If pilots follow their instinct and immediately try to correct a vortex-induced sharp bank, they in practice end up doing so just as the vortex sends them in the opposite direction, making matters much worse. Only when they are out of the vortex should they make corrections.

Added Safety Feature Sometimes Responsible for Disasters

Though there is absolutely no direct link, it is sad to think that in the case of the Asiana A320 that crashed into the Java Sea in 2014, an intermittent fault with the rudder travel limit unit (RTLU), designed specifically to stop pilots doing what Molin did, ultimately led to the disaster.

Due to the fault, that had been occurring on and off for over a year, the captain had to repeatedly reset the system. Exasperated, using a technique a mechanic had taught him that should not have been used in the air, he momentarily switched off a couple of the computers. The autopilot disengaged, and then due to a whole series of blunders and the captain using baffling language the copilot misinterpreted, the aircraft finally stalled and crashed.

---

[1] As explained in connection with the collision between an airliner and a Cessna at Milan's Linate Airport, "runway extension" means the imaginary line that would be drawn if the runway continued.

[2] The NTSB presented a simulated video for the inquiry, showing a side view of the aircraft and the movements of the controls made by Molin.

[3] Four years earlier, the A300-600 pilot of American Airlines Flight 903 lost control at 16,000 feet on approach to Miami and moved the rudder from side to side to recover, almost tearing off the tail in the process.

Subsequently, an Airbus internal memo noted, "Rudder movement from left limit to right limit will produce loads on fin/rear fuselage above ultimate design load." If that memo had been generally circulated, that fact not only might have been incorporated in the AAMP program but mentioned in the manual.

[4] The AAMP program to enable pilots to right aircraft after upsets included aggressive use of the rudder.

Weary Colgan Air Pilots Gossip Before Stall (Buffalo, NY, 2009)

Fifty percent of flights in the US are by regional carriers

> The feeder airline pilots were tired. One was also not very well, and they allowed gossiping to encroach on the time they should have been using to prepare the landing.
>
> Colgan Air Flight 3407, February 12, 2009

Though not a major disaster in terms of the number of lives lost, the Colgan Air Continental Airlines Connection Flight 3407 crash[1] described here received much attention because fatal air crashes in the States had become rare. Another reason was that it made the American public realize how many flights seemingly flown by the majors (with their flight numbers and even their livery) are in fact operated by regional airlines.

Though the Canadian-built Bombardier C4 turboprop airliner[2] used for Flight 3407 had Continental livery, employees of Colgan Air[3] operated and serviced the flight exclusively. Following the accident, legislators passed laws to make purchasers of airline tickets more able to determine on which airline they are actually flying.

Salaries and working conditions at commuter airlines, as opposed to the majors, are less than generous. The forty-seven-year-old male captain and the twenty-four-year-old female first officer, whose gross salary had been $15,800 during the previous year and was less than that of a bus driver, spent much of the flight discussing the difficulties they had in relation to this.

The cockpit voice recorder also recorded the captain stating that he earned a gross salary of about $60,000.

The captain lived in Florida, and the first officer in Washington State, both on the other side of the country from their New Jersey operating base. Both had at one time considered having proper crash pads in New Jersey, but for financial reasons neither had one—there was always the option of resting or sleeping in the crew lounge.

The first officer had come in from Seattle early that morning. She had managed to get a reasonable amount of rest in the crew lounge and on the flight from Seattle but was suffering from a cold and had stated in an exchange prior to takeoff that had circumstances been different she would have called in sick.

She said, "I'm ready to be in the hotel room," to which the captain replied, "I feel bad for you."

Continuing, she went into detail:

> This is one of those times that if I felt like this when I was at home, there's no way I would have come all the way out here. If I call in sick now, I've got to put myself in a hotel until I feel better . . . we'll see how . . . it feels flying. If the pressure's just too much . . . I could always call in tomorrow. At least I'm in a hotel on the company's buck, but we'll see. I'm pretty tough.

The CVR recorded her sniveling and occasionally yawning during the flight.

The captain himself suffered from a sleep deficit built up over several days and could be heard yawning on the CVR. The rest that he had had that morning in less than ideal conditions in the crew lounge could hardly have made up for that deficit.

The flight was to be a short fifty-three-minute hop across New York State to Buffalo, on the edge of Lake Eerie. Near the border with Canada, Buffalo is the second-largest city in New York State, and consequently they were over built-up areas as the aircraft approached the airport.

The CVR recorded the Newark tower controller clearing the airplane for takeoff at about 21:18:23 EST. The first officer acknowledged the clearance, and the captain said:

All right, cleared for takeoff. It's mine.

The intended cruise altitude for the flight was sixteen thousand feet above mean sea level, and the flight data recorder showed that, during the climb to altitude, propeller and airframe deicing were turned on (pitot static deicing had been turned on prior to takeoff) and the autopilot was engaged.

The turboprop reached its cruising altitude of sixteen thousand feet at about 21:34:44. The cruise part of the flight was routine and uneventful, and the only thing remarkable about it was the rapport between the two pilots, which resulted in them indulging in almost continuous nonessential personal conversation.

Although not in conflict with the sterile cockpit rule, which prohibits nonessential conversations within the cockpit during critical phases of flight, as they were above ten thousand feet it did mean that certain tasks, such as checklists, were delayed until the very end of the flight, when they would be busy.

At about 21:53:40 the first officer briefed the captain on the airspeeds for landing, with the flaps at fifteen degrees (Flaps 15), giving 118 knots as the reference landing speed (V_{REF}), and 114 knots as the go-around speed (V_{GA}). The captain acknowledged this information.

Determining the so-called reference speed (for landing) is a key aspect of any landing, as it is the airspeed needed to ensure a stabilized, safe landing. However, the airspeed that the first officer gave was that for normal conditions, not icy conditions, under which, say, an extra twenty knots is added to allow for wings, stabilizers, and control surfaces performing less than optimally.

The flight continued to descend under approach control, with the captain confirming in his briefing the airspeed for the fifteen-degree flaps landing. At about 22:10:23 the first officer asked whether ice had been accumulating on the windshield, and the captain replied that ice was present on his side of the windshield and asked whether ice was present on her windshield side. The first officer responded, "Lots of ice." The captain then stated, "That's the most I've seen—most ice I've seen on the leading edges in a long time. In a while anyway I should say."

About ten seconds later the captain and the first officer began a conversation that was unrelated to their flying duties.

At about 22:12:18 the approach controller cleared the flight crew to descend and maintain 2,300 feet, and the first officer acknowledged the clearance. Afterward, the captain and the first officer performed flight-related duties but also continued the conversation concerning other matters. At about 22:12:44 the approach controller cleared the flight crew to turn left onto a heading of 330 degrees. At about 22:13:25 and 22:13:36 the captain called for the descent and approach checklists respectively, which the first officer performed. At about 22:14:09 the approach controller cleared the flight crew to turn left onto a heading of 310 degrees.

The altitude hold mode became active as the aircraft was approaching the preselected altitude of 2,300 feet, which was reached at about 22:14:30, with the airspeed approximately 180 knots at the time. The captain began to slow the aircraft less than three miles from the outer marker to establish the appropriate airspeed before landing. According to FDR data, the engine power levers were reduced to around forty-two degrees (flight idle was thirty-five degrees) at around 22:16:00, and both engines' torque values were at minimum thrust at about 22:16:02. The approach controller then handed them over to the BUF ATC tower controller. The first officer's acknowledgement of this instruction was the last communication between the flight crew and ATC.

When the first officer, at 22:16:21, told the captain that the gear was down, the airspeed was roughly 145 knots.

The reduced airspeed meant the autopilot had to apply additional pitch trim in the aircraft-nose-up direction to maintain the 2,300-foot altitude. An ice-detected message appeared on the engine display in the cockpit. About the same time the captain called for the flaps to be set to fifteen degrees and for the before-landing checklist. The airspeed was then about 135 knots.

At 22:16:27.4 the CVR recorded a sound similar to the stick shaker. (The stick shaker warns a pilot of an impending wing aerodynamic stall through vibrations on the control column, providing tactile and aural cues.) The CVR also recorded a sound similar to the autopilot disconnect horn, which repeated until the end of the recording.

When the autopilot disengaged, the airspeed had dropped to 131 knots. FDR data showed that 0.4 seconds later the control columns moved aft and that the engine power levers were advanced to about seventy degrees (the rating detent was eighty degrees) a second later. The CVR then recorded a sound similar to increased engine power, and FDR data showed that the engine power had increased to about 75 percent torque.

The stall warning (stick shaker) activates seven knots or so before an actual stall. However, as the reference speed switch on the icing panel had been turned to "Increase," the stick shaker would activate at about twenty knots higher than it otherwise would have done. In addition, the airspeed indicator would have shown the low-speed red markings coming up on the band. Surprisingly, in view of all the talk about icing, the pilots had not even considered increasing their reference landing speed.

The captain had not called out "Stall" when the stick shaker activated, nor had the first officer called out "Positive rate" when the aircraft climbed in response to the captain (presumably) pulling back on his control column. While the increase in power (not to the maximum) could not immediately influence the airspeed, putting the aircraft into a climb certainly did, and it declined rapidly.

After pitching up, the aircraft rolled to the left, reaching a roll angle of forty-five degrees left wing down, and then rolled to the right. As it rolled to the right through wings level, the stick pusher activated as a last resort to prevent a stall at about 22:16:34, at which point Flaps 0 was selected. At about 22:16:37 the first officer told the captain that she had put the flaps up, even though she had not been ordered to do so and in so doing had made recovery from the stall even more difficult, as the aircraft would have to fly even faster in a no-flaps configuration.

FDR data confirmed that the flaps had begun to retract by 22:16:38; at that time the aircraft's airspeed was about a hundred knots. FDR data also showed that the roll angle reached 105 degrees right wing down before the aircraft began to roll back to the left and the stick pusher activated a second time (at about 22:16:40). The aircraft's pitch angle was minus one degree.

At 22:16:42 the CVR recorded the captain making a grunting sound. The roll angle had reached about thirty-five degrees left wing down before the aircraft began to roll again to the right. Afterward, the first officer asked whether she should put the landing gear up, and the captain said, "Gear up" and an expletive. It was too late. The aircraft pitched about twenty-five degrees nose down with a roll angle of a hundred degrees right wing down respectively, with the aircraft entering a steep descent. The stick pusher activated a third time (at about 22:16:50), and two seconds later the FDR data showed that the flaps had retracted fully. About the same time the CVR recorded the captain stating, "We're down," and the sound of a thump.

The aircraft had come down on a single-family home, and a post-crash fire ensued. The death toll was fifty: one person killed in the house, and all forty-nine occupants of the aircraft. The fire, partly augmented by escaping gas from a gas main to the house, destroyed much of the aircraft, making recovery of the bodies and evidence very difficult.

The investigators, as usual, first sought the extremities, such as the nose, wingtips, and tail, to see whether the aircraft had crashed in one piece or broken up before hitting the ground, which it had not. They quickly recovered the FDR and the CVR and found them to be in good condition.

Probable Cause

The NTSB ultimately determined that the probable cause was the captain's inappropriate response to the activation of the stick shaker, which led to an aerodynamic stall, from which the airplane did not recover.

Contributing to the accident were:

1. The flight crew's failure to monitor airspeed in relation to the rising of the low-speed cue.
2. The flight crew's failure to adhere to sterile cockpit procedures.
3. The captain's failure to effectively manage the flight.
4. Colgan Air's inadequate procedures for airspeed selection and management during approaches in conditions where the aircraft would be subject to icing.

There were differing opinions at the NTSB as to how much fatigue was a factor, with some believing it should have been included in the contributing causes. After publication of the official report, a lawyer for families suing over the crash said that newly released e-mails showed Colgan Air doubted the captain's ability to fly the plane six months before it crashed.

These e-mails were not made available to the NTSB in the course of its inquiry. Colgan Air had admitted that it might well not have employed the captain had it been aware of all the checks that he had failed before it engaged him.

The NTSB recommended that there should be a limit to the number of failed checks a pilot is allowed before his or her dismissal. However, the FAA considered this to be too arbitrary and impractical. Yet there have been a number of cases, including a recent Nigerian one, where pilots responsible for crashes have been found to have a checkered history as regards check rides, and with hindsight should perhaps have been let go. Instead of being fired, such pilots are generally sent for remedial training, but one wonders whether any amount of remedial training can make up for a lack of innate aptitude or ability to analyze while under stress.

At one time many commercial pilots in the US came from the military, where the weak ones were quickly weeded out.

Ironically, it was the extra safety feature, namely the special switch for increasing the reference speed setting for icy conditions, that caused the stick shaker to operate and the captain to react perhaps in panic, which bears out the contention of Charles Perrow that safety systems can cause accidents.

The first officer, who was considered to be above average for her level of experience, did not help matters by raising the flaps. Her failure to note the rising low-speed cue with its red markings on the band of the airspeed indicator was attributed to the fact that she was preoccupied with other tasks.

Gossiping had delayed tasks such as checklists. Then the lowering of the flaps and undercarriage would have diverted her attention from the altimeter to the central console.

Of course, the captain should have been monitoring the airspeed himself and picked up on the rise of the red low-speed cue. Could his alleged tendency to rely more than usual on the autopilot to do the flying have got him out of the habit of monitoring airspeed?

His failure to call out "Stall" possibly led to the first officer reacting incorrectly by raising the flaps (to which the captain did not object). To what extent her bad cold and fatigue impaired her monitoring and decision making is difficult to determine.

Sterile Cockpit Rule

This is sometimes cited as an example of what can happen when pilots fail to obey the FAA's sterile cockpit rule, requiring pilots to refrain from nonessential activities, such as idle gossip or unnecessary interaction with cabin crew, during critical phases of flight, in general defined as heights below 10,000 feet (3,048 meters). Passengers will usually hear a chime when the aircraft passes through that 10,000-feet altitude.

---

[1] The previous disaster had similarly involved a commuter airline, the Comair Flight 191 crash in August 2006, where the aircraft with 50 people aboard had taken off on the wrong (much too short) runway. Only the first officer survived, having suffered terrible injuries.

[2] Designed to carry 74 passengers and 4 crew members (2 pilots, 2 cabin crew).

[3] Colgan Air was a regional carrier that flew routes under contract for US Airways, United, and Continental. Pinnacle Airlines Corp, the parent company of Pinnacle Airlines and Colgan Air, filed for bankruptcy protection on April 1, 2012.

Chapter 9
PILOT CRASHES AIRCRAFT INTENTIONALLY?

SilkAir Flight 185 in Near-Vertical Dive (Indonesia, 1997)

NTSB convinced it was suicide; Indonesians unsure

> A US lawyer later managed to sue the makers of the 737's rudder power control unit (PCU), with the jury not permitted by law to consider the NTSB findings.
>
> SilkAir Flight 185, December 19, 1997

The Boeing 737 was the newest in SilkAir's fleet and had been delivered to the airline only ten months before. With ninety-seven passengers and seven crew, it had taken off at 15:37 local time from Jakarta's main international airport, bound for Singapore, a short flight of some eighty minutes.

The captain was forty-one-year-old Tsu Way Ming, a Singaporean, and the first officer twenty-three-year-old New Zealander Duncan Ward.

Before flying commercially, Captain Tsu had been a Skyhawk pilot and Skyhawk squadron instructor in the Singapore Air Force, attaining the rank of major before taking voluntary retirement.

Everything about the flight that day seems normal on the cockpit voice recorder (CVR), with the exchanges between the pilots, and with the cabin crew, nothing out of the ordinary. Neither was there anything strange about the captain's routine address to the passengers over the PA system.

At 15:53 the pilots reported reaching their thirty-five-thousand-feet cruising height, and twelve minutes later, at 16:05, Captain Tsu handed over control to the first officer, saying, "You have the controls," as he absented himself. There was the sound of a seat belt being unbuckled, after which the cockpit voice recorder ceased recording.

Although there was no CVR recording, a routine exchange between the air traffic controller and First Officer Ward was recorded at Jakarta at 16:11, with no indication of anything untoward. However, just over a minute later the controllers' radar showed the aircraft dropping an unbelievable 15,500 feet in just thirty seconds before disappearing from the monitor.

The controllers did not have to wait long for confirmation of the crash, as though in an isolated country area, the scene of the crash was inhabited. There were even eye witnesses who saw the aircraft, having shed some parts, dive almost vertically at terrifying speed into the wide Musi River, near Palembang, Sumatra. There could be no survivors.

Though wreckage was scattered over several kilometers, most of it was in a 200- by 260-foot (60- by 80-meter) area at the river bottom. Because of the force of the impact, the wreckage was in tiny pieces, much of it embedded in the mud.

Not a single complete body or body part was found, since the aircraft and passengers disintegrated on impact. Only six positive identifications were later obtained from the few recovered human remains.

Unbelievably, the whole trajectory, from cruise height at thirty-five thousand feet to impact with the river, took less than a minute.

Powerful dredgers were brought in to scoop up the mud containing the fragments of wreckage in the hope they would include one that could provide a clue as to why the accident had happened. Despite the murkiness of the water, fumbling divers found the flight data recorder only five days after the crash. That, together with the discovery sixteen days later of the bright-orange cockpit voice recorder in the material being dredged up, made the investigators believe the case might be solved relatively quickly.

The Investigation

Apart from the Indonesians, investigators from several countries were involved, and notably the NTSB, from the US. Since the 737 was used in great numbers all over the world, finding any inherent flaw was of great importance.

Unbelievably, 73 percent of the aircraft, albeit in tiny pieces, was recovered. They revealed that the engines were at full power and the controls set to push the nose down rather than up. That alone suggested a pilot might have flown it into the ground on purpose.

However, there had been crashes involving the Boeing 737, described in Chapter 6, where the aircraft had suddenly banked and dived into the ground. It had taken the NTSB years to show that it was due to a malfunction of the rudder power control unit (PCU).

Senior executives of airframe makers, component makers, and engine makers must live in constant fear of waking up one morning to learn something they are responsible for has an inherent flaw, and worse, has caused a disastrous crash. In a scenario that was later to work against them in a US court, Parker Hannifin, the world's largest maker of hydraulic valves, was alerted that radar tracks suggested the accident had something in common with the 737 ones just mentioned, and immediately sent its people out to the site to try to ensure its rudder power control unit (PCU) was recovered.

Retrieved intact, the unit was sent to the US to be checked, and returned, having allegedly been found to be working perfectly—the PCU on the SilkAir 737 was one of the new redesigned ones.

The US's NTSB concluded, after a great deal of painstaking work, that even in the unlikely event of the PCU having caused the upset:

1. The pilots could easily have recovered;
2. The aircraft could not have descended as rapidly as it did without input from a pilot.
   Examination of the debris had shown the engines were at full power, the horizontal stabilizer trim was set at fully forward, and no devices, such as air brakes, were employed to slow the descent.

Other pilots, independently of the NTSB, simulated the descent, and none could achieve such a rapid one without manual input.

Also, the captain could have disabled the CVR—there was a click suggesting he had done so manually on getting up after releasing his seat belt—and later found a pretext for asking the first officer to go back to the passenger cabin, then locked the cockpit door before finally shutting off the FDR. Or he could have struck the first officer on the head. All this would have happened in an ATC no-man's land between that last radio exchange with Jakarta and calling Singapore at PARDI.

On leaving the Singapore Air Force as a major, Tsu had been fast-tracked to the rank of captain at SilkAir, and then to that of line instructor pilot. There were, however, some reservations about his character, and it was thought he needed to be monitored in this respect. In fact, these reservations proved justified, for in the year of the accident he was involved in two incidents.

During a routine approach, which the first officer thought necessitated a go-around because he was too high and too fast, Tsu started weaving to lose height. The "violent rolls, left and right" were, according to the first officer, very disturbing and scary. In the end, they were unable to lose enough height and had to go around. Instead of doing a regulatory conventional one, Tsu did a tight visual circuit at 170 knots within the hills surrounding the airport, with the undercarriage and five units of flap still extended.

As an ex-aerobatics pilot, Captain Tsu probably did not think it amounted to much and failed to report the incident, as required.

Rumors that he was unsafe circulated, and the first officer was asked to submit a report. On the next flight, the two of them were rostered together. Tsu said how displeased he was to hear the rumors about his nearly crashing and about not being suitable for command. The first officer told him he was not the source, which seemed to please Tsu. But just as they began to taxi, he swiveled round in his seat and pulled the CVR circuit breaker, located on a panel behind him. When the first officer objected, Tsu said he had done so to prevent the conversation being overwritten. He wanted to use it as evidence. With the first officer refusing to fly with the CVR disabled, Tsu then said they would return to the terminal to download the recording but changed his mind when the tower asked him to explain why. Tsu then reset the circuit breaker, allowing them to depart. This embarrassing incident, of Tsu's own making, resulted in him being demoted to a mere captain.

There was evidence that Captain Tsu had financial difficulties—his stock exchange trading account had been blocked for nonpayment. However, having sold a couple of properties, he was in fact solvent. What was first seen as a sure sign that it was suicide, namely a life insurance policy starting the day of the flight was later found to have been done to comply with the terms of a mortgage he had taken out. Also, his father was willing to lend him money.

However, the day of the flight did coincide with the anniversary of the day he was involved in an incident where three of his fellow Air Force pilots were killed.

That said, the captain seemed so normal to colleagues, and even in the way he conversed in the cockpit and briefed the passengers.

Also, would one ever kill oneself to claim insurance for one's wife and children on the day the policy started? Doing so would look highly suspicious.

However, the behavior in the cockpit leading to his demotion did suggest an impetuous streak, though the fact that he had asked his wife to meet him at the airport on his return from that flight is seen by some to be proof he was not premeditating suicide before departing.

When the Indonesians produced their final report, they said it was impossible to determine the cause of the crash. This conclusion so infuriated the NTSB investigators who had worked so hard that they added their comments to the report. The investigation had taken three years and left the relatives of the victims angry, and with no closure and a sense of disbelief.

Conclusion

The logical conclusion was that it was suicide, but there was nothing to prove it legally, or behaviorally from Tsu's demeanor in talking to his copilot and particularly the passengers.

Private Investigation and Los Angeles Trial

A US lawyer launched an independent investigation of the recovered rudder power control unit (PCU), and in 2004 a Los Angeles jury ruled that was the cause of the crash. The jury could not be told of the NTSB's findings due to a law designed to ensure the NTSB would come to conclusions without factoring in how they might be used in litigation forbidding it.

Parker Hannifin, the manufacturer of the unit, was ordered to pay US$44 million to the plaintiffs' families. It then appealed the verdict, resulting in an out-of-court settlement for an undisclosed but significant amount. Among the many arguments that helped sway the jury were:

1. Parker Hannifin being immediately alerted thereby suggesting the PCU was potentially suspect,

2. The old flight data recorder that had been installed in place of the solid state one had on that and earlier flights worked intermittently,

3. And if Tsu had switched off the voice recorder why not the flight data recorder at the same time? [The FDR was switched off (or stopped) six minutes after the voice recorder—some suggest when the copilot was out of the cockpit].

One should mention that the lawyer managed to retrieve the PCU from the Indonesians and find an expert to testify as to having found marks suggesting it was at fault, even though Parker Hannifin had not.

Was EgyptAir Flight 990 Revenge? (JFK Outbound, 1999)

Forbidden to fly routes to US due to sexual misconduct

> The US investigators concluded the pilot crashed the aircraft deliberately; the Egyptian side disputed this. Video cameras in the cockpit would have made it possible to prove beyond doubt whether contentious cases were suicides.
>
> EgyptAir Flight 990, October 31, 1999

On board the Boeing 767 EgyptAir flight from New York to Cairo was EgyptAir's chief 767 pilot, Hatem Rushdy. The night before he had told First Officer el-Batouty, who was on board as number two in the relief crew due to take over midflight, that he would no longer be rostered for the flights to the US and it was to be the last such flight.

According to the UK's *Guardian* newspaper dated March 16, 2002, el-Batouty faced ruin following allegations of sexual misconduct, including exposing himself to teenage girls, propositioning hotel maids, and stalking female hotel guests in the US over several years.

Flights to the US came with extra pay besides prestige, so his downgrading and loss of face would be obvious.

Having come from Los Angeles, the EgyptAir 767 lifted off at 1:20 a.m. EST from New York's JFK Airport, where it had stopped to refuel and pick up passengers before continuing on to Cairo.

There were 217 persons on board, including 14 crew, of which four were pilots in two groups—the primary crew and the relief crew.

In the half hour after takeoff, the aircraft climbed to its initial cruising height of thirty-three thousand feet, with flight attendants, and finally Hatem Rushdy, EgyptAir's chief 767 pilot, paying a visit to the cockpit.

After Rushdy left, el-Batouty got up from his seat in the passenger cabin, where he was meant to be resting in readiness for taking over as copilot for the midpart of the flight and entered the cockpit. He then pulled rank, intimating to the much younger primary copilot that they should swap shifts. The latter strongly objected, as it would complicate matters later in the flight and mean he could not rest as planned. Anyway, it was contrary to regulations.

No doubt sensing his close friend el-Batouty's single-minded determination, the primary captain persuaded the younger primary copilot to cede to the older man's demands.

There then followed a routine exchange with the en route air traffic controller, Ann Brennan, who had eight years' experience.

01:47 a.m. ATC:

EgyptAir Nine-ninety change to my frequency one-two-five-point-niner-two.

Captain of EgyptAir 990:

Good day... [Pause while switching frequency] New York, EgyptAir nine zero heavy, good morning.

ATC:

EgyptAir nine-ninety, roger.

Having confirmed they were on the right frequency, Brennan, with her headset still on, moved away from her monitor to deal with paperwork.

When she looked again six minutes later, the echo indicating where EgyptAir 990 should be according to its flight plan was freewheeling because the computers could find no correlation with its transponder. In vain she called them to get them to reset their transponder and tried to contact them through other aircraft and facilities, even asking an Air France aircraft in her zone to fly over them. With it becoming evident something had gone terribly wrong, she, in consultation with her supervisor, set search-and-rescue operations in motion.

The fact that Brennan had not been watching what happened to EgyptAir 990 did not make any difference other than to slightly delay the rescue, when there was no one to rescue, and what she would have seen was recorded anyway and not lost.

What happened in the Cockpit?

At 01:48:03, and shortly after the exchange with air traffic control, the captain announced he was going to the toilet. The aircraft was flying on autopilot at its assigned cruising height of thirty-three thousand feet with no indication of a problem, so it was a reasonable time to do so, for, as he explained, the toilets would be free while the passengers ate their meals. There was the whirring sound of the captain's seat being moved back, followed by the sound of the cockpit door closing.

Then, at 1:48:30, 27 seconds after the captain's announcement he was going to the toilet, there was a muffled sound that sounded like three syllables, with emphasis on the middle one. Despite repeated analysis, the NTSB was never able to grasp what was being said or even determine who was speaking. Some thought it sounded like "Control it" or "Hydraulic."

At 01:48:39, el-Batouty said in a clear but soft voice:

I rely on God! (Tawakkalt ala Allah!)

The significance of these words in Arabic was later to be hotly disputed, with some saying they meant he was going to do something dramatic, and others saying they are words that slip off the tongue easily—when starting your car, for instance.

This was followed by the sound of the whirring of an electric seat and disengagement of the autopilot. If it had disengaged on its own, there would have been an audible warning to alert the pilots.

For four seconds the aircraft flew on, with nothing happening.

"I rely on God," said el-Batouty just as the thrust levers were sharply pulled back to idle. The elevators in the tail that control the pitch of aircraft then moved to the three-degrees-down position. As a result, the nose pitched downward and the aircraft did what is called a bunt, whereby it suddenly pitches so sharply downward that it creates near-zero or negative g.

It is used to throw hijackers off their feet or to get astronauts used to the weightlessness of space flight.

Meanwhile, el-Batouty was repeating "I rely on God" again and again.

The elevators were moved even farther downward, with the pitch of the aircraft attaining forty degrees downward. In the twenty-five seconds from the pulling back of the thrust levers and the movement of the elevators, the aircraft had plunged ten thousand feet, from thirty-three thousand to twenty-three thousand feet, and it was not over.

Almost unbelievably considering the conditions, the captain got back to the cockpit sixteen seconds after the initial pitch down must have made him realize something was wrong. The cockpit voice recorder transcript gives some indication of the situation:

Captain:

What's happening? What's happening?

El-Batouty:

I rely on God.

For about fifteen seconds there were various thumps and clicks, together with a continuous aural master warning, followed by another "I rely on God" from el-Batouty.

Captain:

What's happening?

[unidentified voice]: [unintelligible]
Captain:

What's happening? What's happening?

El-Batouty:

I rely on God.

Captain:

What's happening?

Captain:

What's happening, Gamil? What's happening?

Captain:

What is this? What is this? Did you shut the engine[s]?

Captain:

Get away in the engines. Shut the engines.

El-Batouty:

It's shut.

Captain:

Pull. Pull with me. Pull with me. Pull with me.

The recording ends at 01:50:38 due to lack of electrical power.

Analysis of the flight data recorder data while still working showed the captain, probably standing, had been pulling back on his control column, while el-Batouty had been pushing forward on his, with the unusual result that the left elevator was up and the right one down.

The captain must have had some success in his struggle, for the radar tracks show the 767 leveled out at about sixteen thousand feet and climbed to nineteen thousand, and possibly went as high as twenty-two thousand feet. The recovery and climb only prolonged the agony of all on board, for with el-Batouty having cut the fuel supply to the engines, it would have been impossible to restart them in time even were it possible to subdue him.

The cockpit would have been in darkness, with the sophisticated displays dead and the only light coming from the basic instruments running on battery power.

In the passenger cabins, there would have been light from the emergency lights, including those set in the floor showing the way to the emergency exits.

A major search for survivors was undertaken, but it soon became clear no one could have survived. In a decision they were later to regret, the Egyptian authorities handed over responsibility for the accident investigation to the US, and notably the NTSB, even though the accident occurred over international waters and they had the right to lead the inquiry.

The Investigation

Nine days later the flight data recorder was recovered from the depths and the cockpit voice recorder shortly afterwards. What they revealed was not what the Egyptians expected; instead of an inquiry pointing the finger at a rich foreign entity, such as Boeing, that could be sued, one of their own pilots was likely to blame, bringing shame to their country, and el-Batouty's references to God precipitating a poisonous religious angle, which was played up in the Western press.

What the NTSB thought would be a simple open-and-shut case came to test their patience and waste their experts' time. The Egyptians sent over a team, which installed itself near the NTSB headquarters in Washington, and spent a year coming out with one theory after another as to why, apart from el-Batouty's actions, the aircraft crashed. Each of these had to be checked out. They at one point said it was a cover-up because the US was ashamed at the poor performance of its air traffic control. It was Air Traffic Controller Brennan's fault!

The Egyptian side closed ranks, evidently under orders, making it impossible to get anything other than robotic answers from individuals, whether concerning el-Batouty or the views of their experts.

Though at first sight some of the Egyptians' points may have seemed valid, it beggared belief that the fault in the aircraft they suggested should occur the precise moment el-Batouty found himself alone at the controls. There can be hardly any doubt he crashed the aircraft intentionally.

It seems that revenge, following the conflict with the head 767 pilot, was the principal motive. One might bear in mind that the desire to lay the blame on someone is an element in many suicides.

An article on the ABC News website after the EgyptAir crash said: "Although the actions of the Flight 990 copilot may never be clearly understood, the allegations raise [general] fears about whether pilots may be suffering anything from depression to anxiety, or even a death wish. But are the fears founded? There are, in fact, very few instances in which a pilot's or crew member's deliberate actions are known to have brought down an airplane:

1. In 1982 a Japan Airlines DC-8 approaching Tokyo's Haneda Airport plunged into Tokyo Bay. It was determined that the pilot had pushed the nose of the plane down after fighting off the first officer for control. Twenty-four people were killed and 141 injured. The pilot, who survived and pretended to be a passenger when picked up, was later put into a psychiatric institution.

[Author's note: After this incident, Japanese passengers flying with Japan Airlines would scan the faces of the airline's pilots at the airport for any tic, suggesting mental problems, resulting in the pilots being twitchier than usual.]

2. On August 21, 1994, an Air Morocco jet fell from the sky after its autopilot was disconnected, and fifty-one people were killed. The cockpit voice recorder suggested that the pilot wanted to commit suicide and deliberately crashed the plane.

3. On December 19, 1997, a SilkAir Boeing 737-300 at cruising altitude went into a steep dive after its flight data recorder and cockpit voice recorders had been turned off. It crashed in Palenbang, Indonesia, killing 104 people. The pilot had recently been demoted and was suspected of committing suicide/murder.

4. On October 11, 1999, an Air Botswana pilot, recently grounded for medical reasons, took off in a company plane and threatened to crash it into company headquarters. He ultimately crashed into two other Air Botswana jets on the ground, destroying all three craft and perishing.

5. The closest such American incident involved an off-duty Federal Express pilot, who, while traveling on a FedEx cargo flight on April 7, 1994, attacked the flight crew with a hammer and spear gun in an attempt to take control of the DC-10 and crash it into Federal Express headquarters in Memphis,

Tennessee. The injured flight crew managed to gain control and safely land the airplane.

He had chosen the hammer and spear gun as weapons in the hope that the crash he planned would look like an accident and his family would benefit from the insurance, which would not be the case were a gun found in the wreckage.

To those we must add the more recent Germanwings case.

El-Batouty risking his career through his outlandish behavior in the US brings into question his judgment. He should have been dismissed or given non-flying duties on those grounds alone much earlier.

However, he was a large, popular man three months shy of his mandatory retirement age. Many senior people around him were no doubt aware of his risky behavior but laughed it off, pleased to receive the Viagra he would buy in the US as presents.

Lessons might be learnt from financial institutions, where vast sums of money rather than lives are at stake. There, a dismissed staff member is immediately escorted from the premises. While that may be over the top, when a pilot might feel demeaned, measures might be taken to ensure that he or she is never left alone in the cockpit.

Suicidal Germanwings Pilot Locks Out Captain (French Alps, 2015)

The conundrum of medical confidentiality

> Within two days of the incident there came the shocking news that the aircraft had been crashed intentionally by a pilot with known mental problems.
>
> Germanwings Flight 9525, March 24, 2015

Modern technology in this case allowed some relatives of those on board to follow the flight in real time on Flightradar24 on their smart phones, and they became aware something was wrong as soon as, if not before, the air traffic controllers.

Indeed, one of the first things the French air accident investigators did on finding no transponder returns from Germanwings Flight 9525 and repeated calls to unanswered was to ask Flightradar24 to provide them with its data, which showed the A320 at its cruising height of thirty-eight thousand feet, staying on course toward Germany, but gradually descending, until disappearing sixty-two miles (one hundred kilometers) northwest of Nice.

The air traffic controllers alerted the local mountain rescue team. Almost as if fate had willed it, the first man from the team to be lowered onto the crash site from a helicopter caught sight of an orange box as he, having been told not to touch anything, made his way carefully through the carnage to see whether there were any survivors.

The orange box was the cockpit voice recorder, an item that can take days to find, if ever, and it was to enable investigators to solve the mystery without painstaking examination of every scrap of debris.

Together with the flight data recorder, which was recovered later, it revealed that the first officer, Andreas Lubitz, exploited the captain's bathroom visit by locking him out of the cockpit. He then set the autopilot to the lowest altitude possible, a hundred feet, and calmly waited for the inevitable.

The captain could be heard banging on the cockpit door, pleading to be let in, and even trying to smash it, while Lubitz breathed steadily and was chillingly quiet. Passengers could be heard screaming just before the impact with the mountains.

The flight was a regular Germanwings flight to Dusseldorf that had taken off from Barcelona at 10:01 a.m. local time with 144 passengers and 6 crew. It reached its cruising height of thirty-eight thousand feet at 10:27 while still over the Mediterranean, but as it passed over the French coast near Toulon four minutes later, at 10:31, it began descending and finally hit the mountains ten minutes later, at 10:41.

The inquiry found that Lubitz had similarly toyed with the autopilot height setting on the outbound flight. Whether that was to practice, or whether the captain returned before Lubitz felt fully resolved to go into action, is uncertain.

On the return leg, the toilet next to the cockpit was out of order, forcing the captain to go all the way to the back of the aircraft. It is thought that Lubitz might well have given the captain a diuretic to make him absent himself. Descending even onto mountains from thirty-eight thousand feet takes time, and at various stages Lubitz hastened the descent.

Just before getting up to go to the toilet, the captain told Lubitz to get ready for the landing at Dusseldorf and could not have realized the significance of Lubitz's subsequent comment, which was "Hopefully. We'll see."

Mental Condition

All attention became focused on Lubitz, and when it was found he was being treated for mental problems and had had to take time off from his training at a Lufthansa facility in the US due to depression, anger grew. Doctors knew, and a torn-up sick note for the day of the flight was found in his flat. Germany has very strict laws regarding medical confidentiality, and it was claimed doctors could not have broken it. Even a chit saying someone needs to be off work does not have to indicate the nature of the illness.

In 2009, Lubitz halted his pilot training with Lufthansa, telling friends he was suffering from stress. He was also found to have lied on a FAA form to be approved for flight training in the US, usually a serious offense, but was given a second shot.

A former girlfriend said he admitted receiving psychiatric treatment.

He allegedly told her, "One day I'll do something which will change the whole system, and everyone will know and remember my name."

He had studied modes of suicide on the Internet, and shortly before the flight had gone online to learn how to lock the cockpit door definitively.

According to a doctor treating him, he not only suffered from depression but also from a psychosis that he was losing his sight, when there was nothing wrong with his eyes, and he lived in constant fear of losing his coveted pilot's job, which was everything to him.

Aftermath

The US and China, for instance, already had a rule that there must always be two crew members in the cockpit, and some European countries and airlines immediately followed suit. Lufthansa initially did not but reversed that policy under pressure.

One recommendation was that there should be insurance so that pilots should have some compensation in the event of losing their license and not face what may seem to them ruin.

Chapter 10
UNCONTAINED
ENGINE DISINTEGRATION

"Uncontrollable" DC-10's Miracle Landing (Sioux City, 1989)

Impossible to replicate feat in simulator

> Engines are made of the most advanced materials and their parts are x-rayed for defects so that even twin- as opposed to four-engine airliners can fly miles away from possible landing places.
>
> However, engines can disintegrate, and their parts fly out with tremendous centrifugal forces. This chapter describes two cases where the latter happened, and exceptional airmanship saved the day. Partly in one case, and completely in the other.
>
> United Airlines Flight 232, July 19, 1989

U nited Airlines Flight 232 from Denver to Philadelphia, with a stopover in Chicago, was more than halfway through its first leg. On board the three-engine DC-10 were the two pilots—Captain Haines, aged fifty-seven, and First Officer Records, aged forty-eight—and the flight engineer, Second Officer Dvorak, aged fifty-one, as well as 8 cabin attendants and 285 passengers. It was midafternoon, and they were flying in almost perfect weather at the economical height of 37,000 feet and at their designated cruising speed.

Just as they were effecting a slight change of heading, the aircraft juddered, and passengers heard a thud at the rear.

The instruments indicated something had happened to the number two engine, mounted in the tail, and that it was spooling down. It would have to be shut down in accordance with the engine shutdown checklist, which should be no big problem, as it was the center engine and the aircraft could fly easily on two engines, and especially if the thrust on each side was equal.

While losing one engine was not much reason for concern, much more worrying was the fall in pressure and loss of fluid in all three hydraulic systems. First Officer Records informed the captain that the aircraft was no longer responding to the controls, and on taking over, the captain was able to confirm the desperate situation for himself. Even by deploying the ram air turbine (RAT) to power the emergency generator to supply the backup hydraulic pump, he found it impossible to restore hydraulic pressure. The aircraft was descending slowly, with a gentle rolling and pitching motion.

Minneapolis Center proposed they divert to Des Moines International Airport, which though a hundred nautical miles away had the advantage of wide, long runways. However, the local controller suggested they try Sioux City, as they were already heading in that direction. The DC-10 pilots agreed this was the best option.

With some difficulty they had established direct contact with the company's maintenance department in San Francisco, but no one could come up with any helpful suggestions.

Meanwhile, Captain Fitch[1], a forty-six-year-old off-duty company DC-10 check and training captain, who had been sitting in the first-class passenger cabin, made his presence known and offered his services, which were to prove invaluable as events unfolded.

Captain Haynes asked Fitch to go back to the cabin and check on the damage, and on his return, gave him the task of working the throttles—a key role, as it was the only way they could maneuver the aircraft, and one that would be continuously hands-on. This would leave Haynes and First Officer Records free to deal with the other tasks and, hopefully, find a solution with the help of the airline's experts.

The situation was very similar to that of the Japan Airlines 747 just described in that the DC-10 had what is called a phugoid motion, like a sine wave. On pitching downward, it would progressively gain speed, until at a certain point it would pitch upward and progressively lose speed, until at a certain point it would pitch downward, for the whole cycle to be repeated. The problem was that after each cycle, the aircraft ended up lower, and it would not be long before it struck the ground.

Experimenting with a throttle lever in each hand, Fitch did achieve some measure of control, and finally, by being proactive and anticipating the phugoid motion, was largely able to iron out the highs and lows. The fact that the aircraft had an inherent tendency to yaw to the right and pitch downward, with the right wing tending to drop, made his task even more difficult, as he had to solve the two problems simultaneously. However, one feature that makes the DC-10 easier to control using the engines is that, with the center engine high up at the tail pushing down, the two engines under the wing are very low slung, so that when power is applied to them the nose is levered upward.

Realizing the situation could deteriorate at any moment, Fitch told Captain Haynes they needed to get down as soon as possible. Haynes concurred and asked the first officer to give him the V-speeds for a no-slats, no-flaps landing—they would be able to lower the landing gear using the backup method. The clean—that is, no slats, no flaps—maneuvering speed would be two hundred knots. Furthermore, the speed would have to be above that for Fitch to be able to control the aircraft.

They had dumped fuel, but fifteen tons remained, as the DC-10 has an automatic dump shutoff valve to ensure that dumping cannot reduce the amount of fuel below that level.

The Sioux Gateway Airport[2] controller told them one runway was closed but they could land on either of the other two active runways. Haynes intended to go for Runway 31, which was the longest and widest. However, as they got nearer, Haynes realized that as they could only manage to make right turns and just about manage to fly straight ahead, they could not turn left to line up for an approach to Runway 31.

He asked for, and obtained, permission to go for the closed Runway 22, which by then lay straight ahead. The controller reassured them by saying there would be no trouble with the wind and that the presence of a field at the far end would make up for its shorter length.

The Touchdown and Aircrew Performance

They had no micro-control—that is to say, no means to make last-minute adjustments, such as for the crosswind component—and their speed and rate of descent were extreme to say the least. Maneuvers made by means of control surfaces—that is, ailerons, elevators, and rudder—take effect almost immediately, while control inputs via the throttles have a delay of twenty seconds or even more, depending on what is required. For example, to get into the desired position for touchdown would necessitate preplanned inputs performed some forty seconds beforehand. If something unforeseen occurred, there would be insufficient time to make a correction.

The normal landing speed for a DC-10 is 140 knots, and they were doing 215 knots and accelerating. Worse still, their rate of descent was 1,850 feet per minute and increasing, compared with a normal touchdown rate of descent of no more than 200 to 300 feet per minute. Besides adding an extra ten knots to their landing speed, the quartering tail wind was causing them to drift away from the runway centerline.

Through dexterity and/or good luck, Captains Fitch and Haynes had brought them in almost exactly as intended.

An amateur video (the professional photographers had been expecting the aircraft to come in on the main runway) of the event gives the impression that it is going to be a perfect routine landing.

Captain Haynes[3] has said this video is very deceptive. Though it appears to show them steady at 300 feet, they were losing control and did not have sufficient height to regain it.

The reduction in speed meant the aircraft was commencing a down phugoid and reasserting its tendency to bank to the right. Haynes has also said Captain Fitch, who was at the throttles, added power to correct that bank but that unexpectedly[4] the left engine spooled up faster than the right, making the situation only worse.

The bank increased to twenty degrees, at which point the right wingtip hit the ground just short of the runway and to the left of the centerline, with the nose pointing somewhat downward. The starboard landing gear came down just left of the runway, with the engine on that side striking the ground also to the left of the runway almost at the same time. Accounts then differ.

According to most news reports, the right wing sheared off, and the aircraft flipped on its back, slid down the runway, and then off to the right of it, over a total distance of almost a kilometer. According to Captain Haynes, the aircraft did not cartwheel, as many news reports maintained, but slid sideways on the (intact) left landing gear and the stub of the right wing for two thousand feet.

Finally, the left wing came up, and because there was no weight in the tail, as it had broken off, the aircraft flipped over and bounced.

Examination of the wreckage showed the fuselage had broken into five pieces:

1. The cockpit, where all four occupants survived.
2. The first-class cabin, just behind the cockpit, where, apparently, no one survived.
3. Almost three-quarters of the economy-class cabin, from the front galley behind first-class right back to the trailing edge of the wings, where almost three-quarters survived, albeit with injuries.
4. A short section comprising six rows of seats from the trailing edge of the wings to just before the tail section, where only one person survived, with injuries.
5. The tail section behind that, with just two rows of seats, in which seven people, surprisingly, survived.

Incredibly, 185 people out of 296 survived, making a death toll of 111. That so many survived was to some extent due to the sterling efforts of the cabin crew and their rigorous training in a simulator, which made a crash landing and fire seem real.

Even so, their contribution would have probably been in vain, supposing they were even still alive, had not the high rate of descent and the 215 + 10 knot ground speed been absorbed in some manner.

This is a prime example of the fact that the more horrendous-looking crashes can be the most survivable, due to the fracturing and crumpling absorbing the shock.

Unlike the Staines "heart-attack" crash near London's Heathrow, where the aircraft belly flopped with the landing gear up and the wings level and ended up virtually intact, but with everyone dead or dying, the DC-

10's right wing and right landing gear and right engine struck first and progressively absorbed the downward momentum as they crumpled and sheared off. Then the 3,000-foot skid decelerated the aircraft even more, before the breaking up of the fuselage into five pieces absorbed almost all of what speed remained.

The official report into the accident mentions that the crop of high corn where the main part of the fuselage ended up upside down hampered rescue efforts by firefighters and recommended that having agricultural crops in proximity to runways should be reconsidered.

Thinking of how the rain-sodden ground helped slow Qantas 1 on its 100 mph overrun at Bangkok, one cannot help wondering whether the high corn helped slow the aircraft, or rather, the pieces thereof.

Looking at the feat from a piloting perspective, the main lesson does seem to be the importance of cockpit resource management (CRM), though, according to Captain Haynes, it was first called cockpit leadership management. Each person performed his allotted task and "ideas were thrown around."

With hindsight, one idea that could/should have come to mind was that the pilots transfer fuel from the tanks in the right wing to those on the other side to correct the tendency to bank to the right. Haynes admitted in his presentation at NASA's Dryden Flight Research Center that people would be likely to think of that nowadays, but they did not then, perhaps because they were too preoccupied with immediate problems. One wonders why people back at maintenance did not think of it either.

One problem was that those on the ground took some time to grasp fully what was happening, as the situation was so unbelievable. Certainly, the retention of so much fuel because of the DC-10's fuel dumping restriction was unfortunate—another example of a measure deemed to increase safety doing the opposite.

The Mechanical Causes

The underlying cause of the incident was failure of the engine's fan blade disk due to a casting fault that had remained undetected for seventeen years. The engine had a protective girdle designed to arrest the loss of a single blade flying out prior to the engine being shut down (or spooling down on its own), not to parry multiple blades and heavy fragments of the disk retaining them.

The accident led to much more stringent checks during the manufacture of engine components and during maintenance. In recent years the need to ensure engines are reliable enough for ETOPS has spurred progress in checking such components. The accident also prompted action to find ways of maintaining some measure of control even in the event of such a multiple hydraulic failure.

An interesting point later made by Captain Haynes when giving a talk at NASA's Dryden facility was that modern computers could be made to adapt to flying an aircraft by juggling engine power alone—the pilot would then move the controls in the normal way, and the computer would hopefully do the rest!

Indeed, the FAA and NASA have been looking into this in view of the possibility that airliners will be struck by shoulder-launched missiles, such as happened to the DHL A300 at Baghdad.

Apart from being famous as an exceptional feat of piloting, the Sioux City miracle landing was captured on video and is often shown in documentaries to demonstrate that many survive crashes one would think cannot be survived.

---

[1] Dennis Fitch died of brain cancer on May 7, 2012, aged 69. Many obituaries said how much he was admired as a person and portrayed him as the hero of the Sioux City DC-10 landing.

[2] Sioux City Gateway Airport has the unfortunate three-letter code SUX.

[3] Slide show presentation by Captain Haynes at the NASA Ames Research Center, Dryden Flight Research Facility, Edwards, California (1991).

[4] Just before touchdown, the first officer is telling Fitch to apply left throttle—there seems to be some inconsistency.

Masterful Handling of Stricken A380 (Singapore, 2010)

Shrapnel compromised 95 per cent of systems

> Some in the aviation world said it was not difficult for Qantas to be the "safest airline" (with no hull losses in the jet age), because, unlike the US majors, it mostly flew long-haul routes to safe airports. The edge-of-your-seat incident we now describe shows it perhaps really does deserve the title.
>
> Qantas Flight QF 32, November 4, 2010

Twitter reports said pieces of the aircraft were raining down on Indonesia's Bataan Island. Australians later watching TV even saw footage of locals holding up aircraft pieces, including a large section of an engine cowling with the red markings typical of Qantas livery. Fortunately, no one on the ground was injured or killed, though one piece, still hot, narrowly missed a child at primary school.

Qantas CEO Alan Joyce traveling by car in Sydney with his investment advisers received a phone call asking why the airline's share price was tumbling. His heart sank on being told it was in response to Twitter reports that a Qantas A380 superjumbo had crashed.

Qantas staff raised his spirits somewhat by assuring him that though the aircraft could not be contacted by satellite phone, they were certain it was still airborne, as there had been no report from Singapore air traffic control that it had disappeared from their screens, and Qantas maintenance was as usual receiving telemetric ACARS data (used to report faults automatically before an aircraft lands) from the aircraft.

However, the data was so voluminous that maintenance had initially thought the system itself might be "playing up." Never had they seen anything like it.

QF32

The A380 superjumbo Airbus in question was the first one in the Qantas fleet and named Nancy-Bird Walton after the famous Australian aviatrix. With the flight number QF32, it had taken off on schedule at nine thirty that morning from Singapore, where it had stopped to refuel and allow some passengers to disembark or embark on its almost twenty-two-hour journey from London to Sydney.

The flight was unusual in that in addition to the usual two pilots plus another to allow them to take turns to rest over such a long leg, there were two extra ones, and very senior ones at that. One was an under-training route check captain there to carry out the rostered captain's mandatory annual check, himself being checked by an even more senior check captain.

Too many management pilots in the cockpit in emergencies can spell disaster, and it was good that the rostered captain, Richard de Crespigny, arranged to meet the other two operating pilots beforehand to explain the presence of the check captains and to make clear that he was ultimately in charge, though, of course, following the modern concept of crew resource management (CRM), the captain no longer plays God and considers all views.

The crew's and pilots' flight times were as follows:

1. Richard de Crespigny, captain, and the pilot in command, fifteen thousand hours
2. Matt Hicks, first officer, eleven thousand hours
3. Mark Johnson, second officer, eight thousand hours
4. David Evans, senior check captain, seventeen thousand hours
5. Harry Wubben, route check captain, twenty thousand hours
6. Michael Von Reth, the exceptionally experienced cabin service manager

As customary, the captain sat in the left-hand seat, and the first officer in the right-hand one. Harry Wubben, the route check captain under training himself, insisted on sitting in the middle just behind them, saying that otherwise he could not check on what the captain was doing. De Crespigny was not happy with this arrangement, as to be any use, his second officer should be there. Some tension built up, which Harry Wubben astutely defused by stating he would also assume the role of second officer when required.

On board were 469 people: 440 passengers, 24 cabin crew, and the 5 pilots mentioned.

The leg to Singapore, at almost eight hours, was shorter than the twelve-hour one from London, so the comparatively light A380 did not need a very high thrust setting to lift off easily from Singapore's 4,000-meter (13,123-foot) center runway.

This meant the engines were less stressed than they might otherwise have been and were to be later when climbing under higher power.

It was almost a perfect day as they executed a slight left turn over the sea to take them toward Bataan Island and continued to climb. Apart from having to deviate slightly to avoid ash from a volcano, it looked as though they were in for an easy flight.

Having retracted the flaps and slats to put the aircraft into the clean configuration they would maintain all the way to Sydney, they passed through seven thousand feet on their way to their much higher cruising height, and still gently accelerating.

Moments later there were two bangs in quick succession, which de Crespigny said sounded like a car backfiring. From their instruments, the pilots could see right away it was trouble with the number two engine. De Crespigny immediately set the autopilot to "Altitude Hold," a maneuver he had learnt from a pilot whose 767 suffered an engine disintegration.

It was the quickest way to make the aircraft fly horizontally with reduced thrust in the least demanding way possible, though in fact, with the autothrust surprisingly not working, he had to move the levers himself. He then made a "Pan, Pan, Pan" call to air traffic control in Singapore to signify a serious problem requiring aircraft in their vicinity be kept away, and that as far as possible they not be troubled with ATC demands while they dealt with it.

The passengers were nearer the engine that disintegrated and had heard the bangs and muffled noises more loudly. Not only had the aircraft shuddered, it seemed to them to be falling, but this was an illusion, as by reducing the thrust and leveling off, the captain had abruptly stopped the high-power climb, to which the passengers, with their seatbacks continually pressing firmly against their backs, had become accustomed and which they had come to take as normal.

Pilots are trained to deal with engine failures and even engines falling off, which they are designed to do in certain circumstances, and it is not usually such a big deal, since the aircraft can still fly on those remaining. However, dozens of faults were coming up on the ECAM (electronic centralized aircraft monitor) in addition to the first one, which had been "Engine 2 turbine overheat."

In both training on the simulator and operational flying, the most alerts the monitor would ever show at one time would be two or three. The cabin service manager, who had an unobstructed view of the damage, wanted to tell the pilots how serious it was but found the intercom inoperable.

According to the ECAM, the failed number two engine's thrust had to be reduced to idle and the engine given thirty seconds to settle. It then showed "Fire" before reverting to "Overheat." It was finally shut down and the fire suppressant control selected, but no confirmation that it had functioned was received because the wiring was severed.

These operations were carried out by the first officer with the approval of de Crespigny, who had assumed manual control. The aircraft was flyable but responses to inputs were sluggish. Could the aircraft be gently turned to point back to Singapore's Changi Airport, with its long runways and good emergency services? Gingerly, they executed a wide turn with little bank and found to their relief it could.

Second Officer Mark Johnson was sent back to the passenger cabins to investigate. In first class, right behind the cockpit, he recognized a Qantas second officer traveling back to Sydney, who wasted no time in drawing Johnson's attention to the last thing on his mind, the inflight entertainment system! There on the screen, for all the passengers to see, was a view of the aircraft from a camera high up on the tail, with the left wing punctured by holes and fuel streaming out of the back.

Moving over to the window inset in the left-hand door, Johnson could see what the camera could not, namely the rear cowling of the inside left engine missing and that the inner workings of the engine were exposed. A closer look at the wing revealed a hole so large a man could pass through. Johnson then moved through the cabins, stopping from time to time as "well-placed" passengers drew his attention to disturbing damage. After consulting and briefing the cabin service manager, who needed some info to help him reassure the passengers, he returned to the cockpit, trying to exude confidence he did not feel.

What he had not been able to see was that the fuselage had been penetrated by shrapnel that had severed the two bundles of control wiring which ran up and down it like two spinal cords, making the aircraft paraplegic, as they were to later realize. Fortunately, no passengers had been struck, and at that low altitude the cabin pressure had been virtually equal to the outside pressure, so there had been no explosive decompression, with oxygen masks dropping down.

Now the stream of ECAM warnings made some sense, though the pilots could not know the damage included that to the "spinal cords." The exhausting tasks of dealing with each fault thrown up on the ECAM, and taking appropriate action in consultation with the others, fell to First Officer Matt Hicks.

However, a thought had to be given to the state of the passengers, whom Cabin Service Manager Von Reth had been trying to reassure with the little information he had. Passengers coming off an aircraft safely after a crisis often complain that though the cabin crew did their job, barking orders and telling them to keep calm, the pilots did not tell them anything, not realizing they were too busy saving their lives.

The presence of the extra pilots enabled de Crespigny to delegate that task to Senior Check Captain David Evans, whose calm, measured voice and convincing-but-not-quite-frank words did much to reassure them, and was, according to the quietly confident cabin service manager, Michael Von Reth, the game changer in keeping them under control.

He himself was going through the cabins looking for what are called "ringleaders," people who stand up, go into the aisles or to the doors, and shout "We are going to die!" or similar. Panic is infectious and leads to pandemonium if not nipped in the bud, something that requires psychology and "presence."

Taking Stock and Resolving ECAM Faults

In an aircraft that the pilots knew might at any moment suffer an extra malfunction rendering it virtually if not completely impossible to fly, it took over an hour and a quarter for them to deal with and assess the many faults as best they could and see whether they would be able to land.

The slats on the left wing had been damaged, together with their control systems, and those on both wings had been locked for protection, so they needed to ensure not only that they would have enough low-speed lift and control to land when very much overweight, but also the ability to stop before overrunning the runway, with the fuel very likely catching fire.

Though electrical supply to the left wing had been cut, a fire might still be smoldering there, which was one reason the other pilots opposed de Crespigny's suggestion they climb to ten thousand feet to give them extra height to play with should the three remaining engines they were relying on fail. Besides putting extra strain on the unsure engines, the alteration to the slipstream could possibly exacerbate a fire.

Fuel and its distribution were major problems, as most of the pumps and fuel galleries were inoperable, making it impossible either to move some of the fuel farther forward to adjust the center of gravity or to jettison any. As a result, they were forty-four tons overweight to land. They could not fly around for hours to burn it up, for not only could something else go disastrously wrong, making them lose control, but the longer they flew, the greater the three fuel imbalances between the amount in the left wing, right wing and horizontal stabilizer tanks became. With the right wing already almost eleven tons heavier than the left, limited control of the aircraft meant a difference of much more than that would make them flip over, and particularly at slow speed on landing.

The hydraulics situation was also very worrying. The pressure in the green channel, fed by pumps in the left wing, had fallen to zero, and the yellow one, fed by four pumps driven by engines on the right, was none too healthy; the ECAM was saying two should be shut down, which the pilots hesitated to do as once shut down they could not be restarted. Finally, after some debate they were shut down, with the system seeming okay.

To realize what was involved, and not least the strain under which the pilots must have been, one should read de Crespigny's book *QF32*, still available on Kindle. It also gives a good insight into the complexities of the latest aircraft, which though taken in hand by the computers should ideally be understood by pilots.

In this respect, de Crespigny had the advantage of having studied the complexities while researching a book he was writing, even visiting manufacturers, such as Boeing, Airbus, and Rolls-Royce.

Flying around in a circuit near Singapore, they tried to resolve the almost one hundred problems thrown up by the ECAM, and after they had been solved in one way or another, decided to concentrate on what did work rather than on what did not. Enough was working for the aircraft to fly, but was that sufficient for them to land safely?

They would be coming in faster than usual, and even if they were in one piece on the runway, they might not be able to stop before reaching the end, since there were few spoilers to slow them initially, and they only had about 50 percent braking power, meaning the working brakes would be white hot and liable to set fire to the fuel leaking from the wing. Also, they were considerably overweight, and if they came down hard, the landing gear would collapse, with possibly dire consequences.

They calculated that if all went well and they came in at 166 knots, they could stop with 100 meters (109 yards) to spare. There was a grass overrun area, but there, though the wheels might sink in and slow them, the landing gear might collapse due to their weight, and a fire ensue.

Before making the attempt, and to make it less risky, de Crespigny insisted they perform a control check, something he had experience of in the military, where pilots of aircraft damaged in action had to determine what they could still manage. This in fact simple concept consisted of trying out the landing maneuvers they intended to make high up with enough height to recover—a dress rehearsal of the landing at four thousand feet.

If they found themselves losing control at 166 knots, they would have accelerated and brought the flaps up one step. The point of it was not only to be sure the aircraft would behave under those conditions but also to prevent any speed or stall alarms causing them to react unnecessarily and dangerously. The control checks showed the aircraft could be landed without stalling, though commands would be sluggish.

The Landing

After a long, gentle approach, de Crespigny managed to flare to break their descent and, amazingly, touch down right at the very beginning of the 4,000-meter runway. At the last moment he executed a rarely used counterintuitive maneuver, pushing the sidestick fully forward to make the upwards-facing A380 tip forward. Doing so lifted the low-hanging wheels at the middle and poised the aircraft on a cushion of air, which by virtue of the so-called ground effect helped soften the impact of the overweight superjumbo.

Though four thousand meters of runway lay ahead, the first thousand flashed by with little evidence of slowing, since only limited use of the spoilers and only one engine producing reverse thrust, combined with degraded braking, meant high-speed retardation was poor. Then things started looking better, and they eventually came to a halt just over one hundred meters from the end of the runway.

Being on the ground was in some respects more dangerous than being in the air, for up in the sky the fuel leaking from the wing just disappeared, with nothing hot to ignite it. On the ground it was not only pooling under the aircraft like kindling for a bomb fire, there were also the overheated brakes, with temperatures climbing toward 1,000 degrees Centigrade, that could ignite it at any moment.

With it being the "Kangaroo Route" between the UK and Australia, de Crespigny knew there were many old people, some in wheelchairs, not to mention babies and infants who were liable to be injured coming down the chutes. Once outside, passengers might start a fire with their shoes or mobile phones or might wander to the vicinity of the engine they had been unable to shut down. He therefore did not order an evacuation but told the cabin crew to be constantly ready for one.

Finally, fire crews, who had been holding back due to the unstopped engine, sprayed gallons and gallons of water onto the brakes and covered the fuel with foam. The danger passed as the brakes cooled.

Even so, the passengers had to endure an uncomfortably long wait with no air-conditioning before they were finally allowed to leave without luggage via stairs and were bused to the terminal, where de Crespigny debriefed them.

The care de Crespigny took to look after the passengers, with the help of the other pilots, meant when they eventually faced the press pack on leaving the terminal, they were happy and grateful people and well informed enough not to allow the press to put words into their mouths, such as their aircraft was on fire, which was not the case.

The Extent of the Damage

Close examination on the ground revealed that shrapnel had severed more than 600 wires, including all of one of the "spinal cords" transmitting essential data from systems. The wing had been struck in more than one hundred places, and the fuselage in some two hundred. A heavy chunk of metal had missed the top of the fuselage by inches. Fourteen holes were found in the fuel tanks. Perhaps 95 percent of the systems, including the number one and two AC bus providing essential power for many of them, had failed.

Rolls-Royce

Believing BP made a big mistake by being so open about the Gulf of Mexico oil rig disaster, Rolls-Royce refused to comment publicly regarding the likely cause of the disintegration and how that might have come about, much to the annoyance of Qantas and others. The airline's CEO, Alan Joyce, said BP's mistake lay not in being forthcoming but in saying the wrong things.

The lack of information led to the general impression that Rolls-Royce was running a shoddy, primitive manufacturing operation at the plant where the engine had been made, with poor attention to detail and inappropriate quality control. Though that was partly true, and the issues have since been addressed, the manufacturing and quality control there used very sophisticated equipment.

The error arose from using the wrong datum (reference point) for drilling into the stub pipe to make room for a filter after the object moved slightly; the control check did not reveal the discrepancy, because that wrong datum was again used as reference. The error would have been obvious to the naked eye had the weld at the end of the stub pipe not obscured the cross-sectional view.

According to an Australian investigator, Rolls-Royce had considered the possibility of such a fire but calculated the engine would power down on its own accord rather than speed up—he jocularly remarked the engine was too good! Perhaps this was borne out by the lengthy struggle the firefighters had to shut down the recalcitrant engine, first with water and finally with firefighting foam.

Besides improving manufacturing and quality control, Rolls-Royce have taken measures to ensure such an event cannot have such dire consequences, and this includes software to shut the engine down in such a case. Nevertheless, it is scary to think an engine maker could spend large sums to make fan disks that never should fail—never happened in forty years—and then find some very minor component on the outside could cause one to spin so fast one would.

With Emirates ordering engines from Rolls-Royce for their next batch of A380s, Rolls-Royce's reputation did not appear to suffer irreparable damage, but the financial cost was enormous.

Firstly, they had to replace many of the engines in use by six or so carriers, then not only pay compensation to the insurance company for the A\$139,000,000 it cost to repair the aircraft expensively in Singapore over a period of a year and a half rather than in China, but also compensate Qantas for loss of revenue due to the whole Qantas A380 fleet being grounded.

Outstanding Airmanship

We said fortuitous circumstances made the "The Miracle on the Hudson" possible. To be consistent, we should ask what role luck played here.

Unlike in Sully's case, it was not primordial, but bad luck could have jeopardized everything. Had it been raining heavily, as it so often does in Singapore, perfectly judging the delicate landing, where hitting too hard with a way-overweight aircraft could be fatal, would have been nigh impossible.

Also, with only limited control via the ailerons, a significant crosswind component would have been impossible to counter. A wingtip and then an engine would have snagged the side of the runway, and the aircraft would very likely have spun around and broken up like the DC-10 did at Sioux City after landing with controls taken out following a similar engine disintegration (described in the previous piece). Gusts of wind, as said, could have blown fuel up onto the white-hot brakes and started a fire.

While they were also lucky to have the two highly experienced check captains and a psychologically astute cabin service manager, no one can dispute how well they did and how exceptionally talented they were individually.

Chapter 11
METAL FATIGUE

The Hidden Flaw of the World's First Jetliner (1952 to 1954)

Front-runner falls; others learn

> It does not always pay to be first with a radically new aircraft concept, and the example of Britain's brief stand on the pedestal with the world's first jetliner rather proves that.
>
> BOAC Comet 1 G-ALYZ, October 26, 1952
> Canadian Pacific Airways delivery flight, March 3, 1953
> BOAC Flight 783, May 2, 1953
> BOAC Flight 781, January 10, 1954
> South African Airways Flight 201, April 8, 1954

At the end of the Second World War, and before sky-high taxes made it better to be an accountant than an engineer, the British still expected to be in the forefront of aviation technology and aircraft production. The problem was that while the British had excelled in producing fighters, such as the Spitfire and the Hurricane, the Americans had built up an invincible lead in bombers and heavy transport aircraft that they could switch to work as civilian aircraft at little cost.

With no hope of challenging on that front, the British set about designing an airliner that would exploit a domain where Britain had some sort of lead: jet engines. This would enable them to leapfrog the Americans with an airliner able to fly almost twice as fast.

As the key feature was to be the use of a jet engine, the

government perhaps unfortunately placed its support behind a distinguished aircraft company that produced its own engines—the de Havilland company, maker of the famous all-wood Mosquito, as well as the later Vampire jet fighter.

The major concern from the design point of view was conceiving an airliner that would handle well on takeoff and landing, as well as at the much higher cruising speeds contemplated. Not enough thought was given to the fact that flying an airliner at thirty-five thousand feet or more put it in a completely different category as regards pressurization and the effects thereof, and notably metal fatigue of which not so much was known at the time.

Passengers do not require cabin pressure to be the same as that on the ground, but for them to be comfortable, it should not be lower than that at about seven thousand feet, a height at which even people with asthma are comfortable.

For post–Second World War piston-engine airliners, such as the very successful and beautiful Lockheed Constellation, cruising at twenty-one thousand feet, having the cabin pressure equivalent to that at seven thousand feet, meant the pressure difference between the inside and outside corresponded to fourteen thousand feet. The pressure difference for a jet, such as the Comet, cruising at thirty-five thousand feet would be double that: twenty-eight thousand feet!

In addition, there is a world of difference between a fighter with no passenger cabin and an airliner destined to carry dozens of passengers. Indeed, it took de

Havilland four years to get a prototype into the air and two and half years more to have a certified aircraft. A limited scheduled service between London and South Africa finally began on May 2, 1952.

With airlines worldwide showing keen interest, de Havilland soon realized its jetliner should have been larger and proposed a Comet 2, followed by an even larger Comet 3 for what should have been highly profitable transatlantic services. Affluent passengers were boasting about their flights, not only stressing their speed but also their comfort and smoothness.

The First Accident (No Fatalities)

On October 26, 1952, less than six months after the start of commercial flights, the first mishap occurred. A Comet taking off in rain at night from Rome's international airport with a full complement of passengers started juddering and buffeting just as it was reaching the rotation speed (V_R) of around 112 knots. Sensing the aircraft was stalling and would not gain enough speed, the captain pushed the control column forward but, finding that did not solve the problem, cut the engines and applied maximum braking.

The aircraft exited the end of the runway at high speed and ended up some distance away, with the landing gear ripped off and fuel leaking onto the ground from a ruptured fuel tank. Fortunately, there was no fire and all the occupants survived—very shocked but unscathed. The aircraft was a write-off.

Somewhat like the Qantas overrun at Bangkok, the absence of fatalities or even injuries meant the incident received little publicity. The Italian investigators did not even publish their report. Having found marks on the runway showing the tail had struck it a number of times even before reaching the point where the aircraft would normally rotate for takeoff, the investigators concluded it was not the aircraft's fault but the pilots' for prematurely raising the nose on the takeoff run.

Group Captain John Cunningham, de Havilland's famous chief test pilot, carried out tests that showed raising the nose too early increased drag so much that the aircraft could never reach takeoff speed. One wonders whether this shortcoming was not in part due to de Havilland previously working mainly in designing fighters with surplus power, where a tiresome quirk like that would not matter.

Early jet engines did not have the abundant power they have today, enabling aircraft to soar into the sky. They were not much different from piston-engine aircraft, such as the Lockheed Constellation, which to the author seemed to take off like swans, with their "flippers flicking over the water's surface." Manufacturers had not yet fully considered exploiting leading-edge devices able to give considerable extra lift without excessive drag at low speeds. Even the early Boeing 707-100s that stepped into the Comet's shoes only had partial slats inboard of the outboard engine pylon. Full-wing slats only came in later versions.

All Comet pilots were told to keep the nose down until reaching takeoff speed, but with no dedicated attitude indicator showing the attitude in degrees, any abnormal nose-up attitude proved difficult to detect when concentrating on the runway ahead and occasionally glancing at an artificial horizon, which would only give a rough indication. In addition, the hydraulic controls of the day did not simulate a feel, and the pilots could be pushing the tail down with the elevators without realizing it.

The Second Accident

When the first of three Comets ordered by Canadian Pacific Airlines was ready for delivery early in 1953, de Havilland persuaded the Canadians to have it delivered via Australia. This would provide a chance to demonstrate it Down Under and produce worldwide publicity if they could break the record for the time taken to fly from England to Australia in the process.

The aircraft took off from England on March 2 with a five-man flight crew headed by Canadian Pacific's overseas operations manager, Captain Pentland, who in his administrative role had little experience of flying the Comet and had never taken off at night at its controls.

Early the next morning, and while still dark, the Comet was taking off from Karachi at its maximum permissible takeoff weight, only to find the Rome scenario repeated but with a less favorable outcome.

After failing to lift off either on the runway or on the 180-meter overrun, the Comet exploded on encountering several obstacles situated beyond.

The five-man crew and six de Havilland technicians, who were traveling as passengers and were going to assist Canadian Pacific with the aircraft, were killed.

Again, witnesses noted the unusually high nose-up attitude maintained for most of the takeoff run. Just as at Rome, the runway marks showed the tailskid had scraped the runway at several points. It seemed the pilots corrected the nose-up attitude at the last moment and almost succeeded in lifting off.

Investigators concluded that fatigue and pressure to beat the record had been contributing factors in what they classed as "pilot error."

Canadian Pacific immediately canceled its order for the two aircraft de Havilland was prepping for delivery. The accident was bad publicity for de Havilland, but it could still attribute it to pilot error and argue that with some modifications and better training there should be no more such silly accidents. It was fortunate that up to then the number of fatalities had been mercifully small.

The Third Accident

The Comet bound for Delhi had taken off from Calcutta midafternoon on May 2, 1953. There had been no problem lifting off, as the aircraft was quite light, with a crew of six and thirty-seven passengers, and only the fuel required for the two-and-half-hour leg to Delhi.

Twelve minutes after takeoff, the crew duly reported to Calcutta that they were climbing to thirty-two thousand feet, before calling the controller at Delhi, who replied without getting a response. Repeated efforts failed to get any response, and nothing more was heard radio-wise from the aircraft.

Witnesses later reported hearing a bang during an exceptionally severe thunderstorm and seeing a blaze in the sky around that time and at the location of the aircraft.

The aircraft had, in fact, disintegrated in midair. Based on evidence that the horizontal stabilizer had failed due to an exceptional downward force, an Indian High Court judge concluded the accident was due to the storm, and that any aircraft would have broken up in the same circumstances.

Experts reexamining the debris in England drew the same conclusion. They thought it possible the lack of feel in the controls had led the pilots to overcontrol, especially as the captain had for much of his career flown flying boats, where heavy control inputs were the norm.

It was thought the explosive decompression (presumed to have followed separation of the tail fin) occurred as the aircraft was climbing through twenty-seven thousand feet.

People were getting apprehensive, but there was no proof that there was anything inherently wrong with the aircraft itself. The eight accident-free months that followed seemed to confirm this.

The Fourth Accident

Then, on January 10, 1954, a Comet inexplicably disintegrated in midair south of the Italian island of Elba.

The aircraft with six crew—in those days the pilot and first officer were complemented by an engineer and radio officer—and twenty-nine passengers had taken off from Rome for London on the last leg of the run from Singapore. The fact that the aircraft had disintegrated in midair probably while climbing through twenty-seven thousand feet, just as in the Indian case, was thought to be a coincidence.

De Havilland had tested the Comet's cabin under high air pressures and severe conditions prior to production and concluded that it should have been able to withstand fifteen times more flights than the 1,200 that the aircraft had done. The Comets were withdrawn from service for modifications made on the basis that the cause was most likely an in-flight fire or engine fan blade separation.

The Fifth Accident

Eleven weeks after the Elba accident, the Comets were put back into service, only for yet another inexplicable accident to occur two weeks later. Again, the aircraft happened to have taken off from Rome. It was the evening of April 8, 1954.

The Comet in question was one leased to South African Airways and crewed by staff from that company. With only fourteen passengers, the flight can hardly have been a profitable one—memories of the Elba accident had no doubt dampened people's enthusiasm.

The pilots reported to Rome they were climbing to its cruising height of thirty-five thousand feet and seven minutes later called Cairo to report their ETA, after which nothing more was heard of them. The aircraft had disintegrated twenty nautical miles off the Italian coast, southeast of Naples. It had occurred at roughly the same time after departure and at a similar height to the previous one, off Elba.

With Britain's dream shattered, the aircraft's Certificate of Airworthiness was withdrawn. Until the exact cause of the disasters could be definitively determined, and adequate steps taken to prevent any chance of a re-occurrence, the Comet bandwagon was halted in its tracks.

Testing to Destruction in Water Tank

Prime Minister Churchill ordered that everything should be done to resolve the matter, including testing of the fuselage to destruction in a water tank pressurized and depressurized repeatedly to simulate actual flights.

The wreckage of the last disaster had fallen in such deep water that little could be done to recover it with the technology available at the time. However, the Elba wreckage was more accessible, and a crucial piece of evidence was recovered: the tail, with paint marks on it indicating it had been hit by a passenger seat ejected from the cabin, which could well have happened due to a pressurization failure of the cabin. In late June, the fuselage undergoing testing in the water tank finally failed at a rivet hole adjoining one of the square escape hatches. More detailed inspection revealed fatigue cracks that could have been the failure point in rivet holes in the vicinity of the cutout for the ADF antenna in the roof of the cabin.

If the failure had not occurred at the escape hatch, which had been recovered intact, it in all likelihood would have occurred in the vicinity of the ADF cutout. Assuming the failure had occurred there, they tried to work out where the part in question would have fallen, and finally recovered it. The telltale fatigue cracks were duly found, and they had the definitive answer they wanted.

The five remaining Comet 1s had become junk, and a number of Comet 2s in the course of production were modified and bought by Britain's Royal Air Force. They had a heavier-gage fuselage, the safer round, smaller windows, and with the RAF operating them at a slightly reduced cabin pressure gave good service for many years without any serious problems.

Hopes Dashed Again

In October 1958, more than six years after the first scheduled Comet service to South Africa, BOAC launched a transatlantic one with the larger, radically redesigned and strengthened Comet 4s. However, what was to be the Comet's second honeymoon was cut short three weeks later by the arrival of Boeing's much larger 707, with its longer range, greater speed, and greater economy, developed in tandem with the KC-135 air refueling tanker funded by the US Air Force Strategic Command.

Flexing Aloha 737 Lands with Passengers Exposed (Hawaii, 1988)

Famous photo showing passengers exposed to elements

> In the 737, Boeing designed the fuselage so in the event of a failure a structural flap would open to release the cabin air without destroying the structure. Unfortunately, when the failure occurred on Aloha Flight 243, the updraft sucked a female flight attendant standing below up into the aperture, plugging it, with the result that a large section of the roof separated.
>
> Aloha Airlines Flight 243, April 28, 1988

U sed for inter-island hops, the eighteen-year-old Boeing 737 had 89,680 cycles to its credit, or rather, debit. Dividing the hours it had been airborne by the number of cycles, the average flight time worked out as twenty-five minutes.

Only one other 737 in the world had as many cycles.

Admittedly, the impact of these cycles on the structure was in theory less than usual in that the aircraft would hardly ever reach great cruising heights. On the other hand, they were operating in and parked in the warm, salty, and humid environment associated with the Hawaiian Islands in which metal easily corrodes.

Furthermore, the airline operated within tight financial constraints and extracted the most from its geriatric fleet by doing important fuselage checks piecemeal overnight, it being imperative to have the aircraft back in the sky early the next day.

Some operations, such as checking rivets and the bonds holding the fuselage together, require not only very diligent and tedious work but also setting up gantries and safety harnesses if upper parts of the fuselage are to be checked safely, all limiting the effective inspection time. Worst of all, workers suffering from upset sleep rhythms can very easily miss defective areas perhaps in poor artificial light.

In fact, on boarding in the good light of the early afternoon, one of the passengers noticed a small horizontal crack along a line of rivets to the right of the forward left-hand door and had even thought of reporting it to the crew but did not do so for fear of being thought foolish.

The aircraft was already making its ninth flight of the day, this time the thirty-five-minute leg from Hawaii's Big Island (Ito) to Honolulu, on Oahu Island. Its route would take it close to several other islands in the Hawaiian chain, including Maui.

Twenty minutes after takeoff, it had leveled out at its cruising height of twenty-four thousand feet, with thirty-seven-year-old First Officer Madeline (Mimi) Tompkins at the controls. She had eight thousand hours' flight experience and hoped soon to be promoted to the rank of captain, like Captain Schornsteimer, sitting next to her, who had a similar amount of flying experience.

A loud bang behind the pilots signaled the beginning of an explosive decompression. Tompkins later said the decompression was so rapid that the displacement of the small amount of air in front of her was enough to throw her head back.

Donning their oxygen masks according to regulations, with the captain taking over control, as is usual in an emergency, the two pilots tried to assess the situation.

Glancing behind him, Schornsteimer was shocked to see some blue sky through the doorway where the blown-off flight deck door had once been.

Had he been able to see the full extent of the damage, he might not have made such a rapid emergency descent, with the airspeed attaining 280 to 290 knots even with deployment of the air brakes. This is standard practice in the case of a decompression, so the passengers can breathe more easily, but is contraindicated when doing so might lead to the structural breakup of the aircraft.

Having seen the sky through the cockpit doorway, the captain would have realized some passengers would not have oxygen masks, and he felt a rapid descent was necessary for their benefit. He could not see enough to realize that with so much of the upper fuselage missing, he was exposing them to a vicious slipstream and, worse, going so fast could bring about the breakup of the structurally impaired aircraft. Schornsteimer later received many plaudits for his airmanship but was criticized by the investigators on this point.

As the aircraft slowed at a height where breathing was easier for all, the plight of the eighty-nine terrified passengers and the remaining two female cabin attendants became more bearable.

Some had seen the shocking sight of Flight Attendant Clarabelle Lansing, who had been working at the airline for thirty-seven years, sucked upward into a hole (the safety flap) that opened up in the left of the roof near row five, before the whole section around it came away.

Another flight attendant, Jane Sato-Tomita, who had been standing three rows farther forward, not far from the flight deck door, had been severely injured by flying debris and, notably, that missing cockpit door. The other flight attendant, Michelle Honda, had been thrown about and suffered bruising but, being much farther back, in the part of the cabin that still had a roof, was relatively unscathed. Dragging herself on her hands and knees up the aisle against the slipstream, she had to shout in passengers' ears to communicate. Unable to contact the flight crew over the intercom, she at one moment thought the pilots might be incapacitated and asked likely prospects whether any of them could fly a plane.

Unlike the flight attendants standing in the forward part of the aircraft briskly serving drinks in the little time available before their expected arrival at Honolulu, the seated passengers there had seat belts to save them from serious injury or even death.

The pilots, who were very much alive and the least subject to the elements, found the aircraft was controllable, albeit somewhat abnormally. Apart from the distortion of the airflow over the fuselage caused by the gap, the nose was in fact drooping down about a meter below where it should have been and springing up and down.

Some maintained only the seat-fixation rails running longitudinally along the cabin floor were holding the aircraft together—hence the springiness.

The pilots decided to divert to Maui's Kahului Airport, by then only some twenty nautical miles away. This was on the opposite side of the island and involved an approach between two high mountains, which, though not inherently difficult, could have been fraught with danger for an aircraft in its condition, as the violent wind and turbulence could easily break the fuselage apart. Luckily, the wind was much weaker than usual.

Their immediate problem was radio communication, largely due to the wind noise, which made it virtually impossible to hear or be heard. It took some time even for the Maui controller to get their flight number right and then to grasp the seriousness of their predicament, of which even the first officer, handling the radio, was unaware, as she had no intercom contact with the passenger cabin and had to assist the captain. Maui ATC asked them to switch frequencies, as if it were a normal flight.

The investigators criticized this obligation to change radio frequency on the grounds that aircrew dealing with an emergency should not be distracted by this task, which had the added risk that contact with the aircraft might be lost altogether. This reminds one of the criticisms leveled at ATC in connection with the famous crash of a 737 at Kegworth in the UK the following year, where the pilots shut down the good engine instead of the bad one and, incidentally, had to hop from frequency to frequency. A call from air traffic control interrupted their review of the situation.

On lowering the landing gear, the pilots found there was no green light to confirm the front nose wheel was down and locked. Fearful that the aircraft would break up if they delayed, they decided to forgo the usual procedure of overflying the airport for the tower to make a visual check, which would entail a circuit to bring them back to the touchdown approach. The captain decided to come in anyway.

As they came in, the control tower was able to confirm the front wheel was down but obviously could not be sure it was locked.

When the amount of flap was increased to fifteen degrees for the landing, the aircraft began to misbehave, and the setting was quickly reset for five degrees, with the first officer having to consult her manual and make quick calculations to work out the V_{REF} (landing airspeed) for that configuration, which was 152 knots. However, finding the aircraft unstable at that speed, the captain opted for 170 knots, but as he moved the throttles the port engine failed and would not relight.

With the other engine he was still able to bring the aircraft in at the higher speed, telling the first officer, who suggested increasing the flaps to forty degrees detent at the last moment, to wait until they were on the ground before doing so.

Despite or thanks to the higher than usual speed, the aircraft touched down smoothly, with the nose wheel holding. Observers saw the fuselage flexing as if it might snap at any moment. Using the brakes and reverse thrust on the operable starboard engine, the captain successfully brought the aircraft to a halt on the 6,995-foot (2,133-meter) main runway.

It was only after shutting everything down and moving back to assist with the evacuation that the pilots realized how close they had been to the aircraft snapping in half at any time or tearing itself apart during their rapid descent to a level where passengers could breathe without masks. With no upper fuselage to take the compressive forces, the fuselage could have snapped upward at the last moment had they come down too hard on the nose-wheel. It is not clear whether anyone has mentioned that the lack of a green to confirm the nose-wheel was locked might have made the captain more careful than he would have been to bring the nose down gently and may have been a blessing in disguise.

Effect on Passengers

The only passengers unscathed, apart from eardrum problems, were those sitting right at the rear of the passenger cabin, which retained its roof. Those immediately behind the break were hit by debris and suffering from lacerations, often to the face.

Worst affected were those sitting in the area exposed to the elements, some of whom were trapped in their seats in places where the floor had buckled upward beneath them due to the air pressure in the hold below.

Those able to vacate their seats and walk either evacuated via the stairs at the rear or the emergency slide at the main door at the front, with at least one dithering passenger having to be pushed onto the slide by the first officer.

The fire crew was able to extract and evacuate the others in less than half an hour and dispatch them to hospital by ambulance.

There were a whole range of major and minor injuries, including lacerations from flailing wires and even electrical burns caused by contact with them. It took time and therapy for some to recover psychologically from what must have been a very scary experience.

Search of the ocean where the explosive decompression had occurred failed to produce either the body of the ejected flight attendant or any useful material evidence.

The Investigation

With key evidence missing, investigators had to work out what had happened from cracks and disbonding on the periphery of the hole.

Also, to understand the conclusions of the investigators, one needs to know how the fuselage of those early 737s was assembled or, rather, riveted and glued together, and remember that to save weight, the skin of an airliner is often only the thickness of a credit card. Even the thickness of the paint or lack thereof can make quite a difference to the overall weight.

The fuselage consists of overlapping panels mounted on a frame and riveted together. However, unlike a ship's hull, where the rivets can hold the thick plates together with tremendous force, rivets holding the outer skin of an airliner can only get a limited purchase, as they have to be countersunk to ensure a clean airflow over them.

If subjected to repeated stresses, cracks develop in the skin around them.

Therefore, Boeing and other manufacturers decided to bond the overlaps with epoxy resin, in principle using the rivets solely to hold the surfaces together while the resin cured (set) and bonded the joint. Of course, the rivets would provide residual strength to the joint in the event of failure of the bond and allow time to discover the problem during maintenance.

As many who have used epoxy glues know, mixing the two resins together in the right quantities with adequate mixing every time is no easy task. Boeing thought it had solved the problem by putting the mix on a scrim tape. Kept in a refrigerator to prevent curing, the tape would be used as needed and sandwiched between the overlaps before riveting. In theory, it should have produced a perfect bond, but in practice this was not always true for a number of reasons, including dirt and humidity.

If an aircraft is being operated in a hot, salty, and damp environment, corrosion in the poorly bonded areas can push the bonded parts apart, so that they in turn disbond until only the rivets are holding the assemblies together. Then, with all the stress and weakness concentrated along that line, a long crack can result.

Boeing was aware of the problems associated with the bonding in the earlier models of the 737 but largely dismissed the possibility of a failure leading to a catastrophe, as it had devised a safety flap system. This consisted of having the skin crisscrossed by tear straps that would arrest and divert any crack that was actually opening up (called the lead crack) at right angles, thus creating a triangular flap that would blow out and relieve the pressure before further damage was done. These tear straps created ten-inch squares, big enough to relieve the pressure but not so big as to significantly weaken the structure in the process. Not everyone agreed this would work, thinking it might not save the situation in the event of a crack along a line of rivets extending over several potential flaps.

From evidence from the passenger mentioned above and signs of a crack on the same horizontal line of rivets on either side of the gap, the NTSB investigators concluded that this was what had indeed happened.

Theory That Ejected Flight Attendant Plugged Flap

They later accepted as theoretically possible but unlikely a scenario put forward by Matt Austin, an engineer specializing in pressure vessel explosions, which suggested that the safety flap mechanism did initially work as intended but subsequently failed because the lost flight attendant, Clarabelle Lansing, was sucked into it in the process.

Austin was basing this on his experience of pressure vessels, where an initial rupture can be forced wide apart by a fluid hammer effect when debris, for example, blocks the orifice, the powerful hammer effect around the hole being similar to that produced when one replaces the plug in one's bath while water is still flowing out.

According to Austin, Clarabelle Lansing was the plug. There is certainly some evidence that that was what happened, as some passengers saw her being sucked leftward and up into an opening. Signs of blood spatter found (possibly seen in photos) on the remaining part of the fuselage aft of that point seem to be a good indication that she was caught there for a moment. If she had gone straight out as the roof opened up, there would not have been any blood.

However, the NTSB's investigators stood by their initial findings as to the trigger for the failure, and their recommendations remain valid. Adding such grisly details would not change much. Should they have recommended that safety flaps be considerably larger than just ten inches square? Tests might show that the individual would have to be standing up and wearing a skirt to be sucked sideways and up into the venting flap.

Rethink Regarding Aging Aircraft

The Aloha incident had a galvanizing effect in aviation circles, with the realization that many had been complacent regarding aging aircraft. Outside those circles, the pictures of the roof of an airliner blowing away as if it were a tent in the wind produced tremendous pressure from both the public and the media on Congress, which in turn pressured the FAA, with the threat that if nothing was done, aircraft over a certain age would be banned outright.

The Aloha incident and subsequent accidents had the beneficial effect of getting Congress to fund the employment of additional FAA field inspectors, their number having dwindled from 1,672 to a low of 1,331 in 1984 despite the need for more stringent checks to prevent airlines cutting corners to maintain profitability in the face of deregulation.

One problem was that the airlines were not following the directives and advice provided by the manufacturers and the FAA. In their defense, one should point out that the FAA had drafted its directives in something resembling legalese and that a small airline like Aloha would have needed someone to translate these into a form the mechanics could grasp.

Many said some other airlines were as bad, and that Aloha was merely the first to have a failure because their old, high-cycle aircraft were operating in the particularly hot, salty, and humid environment in the Hawaiian Islands.

The incident and the strained relations with John Maple, the principal maintenance inspector, assigned by the FAA to Aloha, made Boeing rethink its confidentiality policy. Boeing, thinking like medical doctors, felt that patients might hesitate to come to them with problems if they thought they would be reported to the regulators.

FAA inspector Maple, who said he had prompted Aloha to get Boeing to review its maintenance procedures, was furious to find himself excluded from the meeting at which Boeing reported the results. Since then Boeing has told airlines to report problems themselves, as it will do so anyway.

Boeing might have been justified in its thinking about confidentiality, but now, with lawyers avid to find any cover-up and sue, the downside risk of that informal approach is probably too great anyway.

Although not in any of the official reports, it is alleged Boeing staff traveling as passengers on the aircraft in question felt it was in a pretty bad way due to the rattles, as did another frequent traveler, who said it felt like an old car.

The excellent article by Martin Aubury in the BASI journal from which some of the information here is drawn finishes by saying the teams setting out to investigate the problems with aging aircraft concluded that checking the obvious was not enough, and that:

1. If signs of corrosion are found, it must be assumed the state of the whole aircraft is questionable;

2. If a problem is found, a proper fix is essential. Repairs are sometimes badly done, with questionable techniques. These probably seem strong at the beginning but may fail later, as happened in the case of the repairs to the aft pressure bulkhead in the JAL 747, which resulted in the worst single-aircraft disaster ever.

3. A repair making one part too strong may produce stress elsewhere. In addition, repairs may hide other defects or make them difficult to see. They therefore need especially careful and thorough checking.

Aftermath

The incident made airlines all over the world and the FAA and other overseers bring in stricter regulations regarding periodic checks of old aircraft. These checks are time-consuming and expensive and are why some airlines prefer to dispose of their older aircraft earlier rather than later.

Chapter 12
TURBULENCE, ICE,
AND WIND SHEAR

Sightseeing BOAC 707 Breaks Up (Mount Fuji, Japan, 1966)

With no FDR, tourist's movie camera was key evidence

> When flying still had something of the frontier spirit
> about it, a BOAC captain might sometimes offer his
> passengers a treat. What better treat could there be than
> giving them a close-up view of Japan's renowned Mount
> Fuji?
>
> BOAC Flight 911, March 5, 1966

W eather conditions that day were so good that from Tokyo one could clearly see the ice-capped cone of 12,390-foot Mount Fuji some eighty kilometers or more away. This prompted the captain of the British Overseas Airways Corporation (BOAC) flight to Hong Kong to change his flight plan at the last minute.

Instead of the usual Jet Green 6 airway, from Tokyo's Haneda Airport out over the sea to Oshima Island and on to Kagoshima in the south, he would take the scenic overland Red 23 airway, skirting Mount Fuji and onward to the industrial city of Nagoya.

The seventy-five-strong American tour group he had on board would surely be highly appreciative.

Despite the bright sky overhead, the atmosphere at Haneda Airport was more than somber.

Only a month earlier an All Nippon Airways Boeing 727 had crashed fifteen kilometers away from the airport. As if that had not been enough, the previous night, with many aircraft diverting due to visibility just below the one-kilometer minimum, a Canadian Pacific DC-8, whose captain was determined to land there, had circled for forty-five minutes, until visibility improved just enough for him to be allowed to make an attempt.

In their haste to seize the opportunity before the weather closed in again, the pilots of the DC-8 descended too steeply. The tower told them they were too low for the distance they were from the runway and instructed them to abort the landing. Disregarding this, the pilot continued, his aircraft first snapping off a number of the frail posts set in the sea to support the approach lights before smashing into the unforgiving concrete of the airport perimeter sea wall.

Only eight of the seventy-two occupants survived the ensuing blaze.

The next day the pilots and passengers of the BOAC Hong Kong flight could hardly have failed to gaze at the charred debris of that DC-8 as they turned onto the runway to line up for their takeoff for Hong Kong. According to some perhaps over-imaginative Japanese newspapers, this horrific sight might have contributed in some way to the deadly accident that was to befall the BOAC flight, in that it must have unnerved the pilots.

Leaving the charred debris behind, the BOAC 707 lifted off and made a wide turn to join the Red 23 airway.

On reaching almost seventeen thousand feet, rather than continuing his climb to cruising height, the captain initiated a gradual descent. Then in what must surely have been an intended deviation from the airway that for safety reasons skirted Mount Fuji, the aircraft apparently veered from a heading of 246 degrees to a heading of 298 degrees magnetic, taking it toward the conical peak of the mountain, only some ten miles distant. Possibly the captain intended to "snake" so passengers on both sides would get a view without rushing to one side and possibly risking upsetting the aircraft.

Just as the passengers were about to get the wonderful close-up view of the mountain, a violent force of air pushed the vertical tail fin (vertical stabilizer) so sharply to the left that it broke off, taking the horizontal stabilizer on the left-hand side with it. This, possibly with the help of the violent air turbulence, destabilized the aircraft, so that shock of the airstream striking it obliquely immediately made it break up.

People below could see it falling from the sky, trailing vaporized fuel, thought by many to be smoke. Some even took photographs. No Mayday call or any other radio transmission was made.

Authorities diverted a US Navy A-4 fighter from the nearby Atsugi air base to look for signs of wreckage. It encountered such violent turbulence in the area that the pilot almost lost his own craft.

According to Macarthur Job (*Air Disaster*: *Vol. 1*), the navy pilot said afterward, "I flew into the same turbulence and truly thought the airplane was going to come unglued . . . My oxygen mask was pulled loose, my head was banging on both sides of the cockpit canopy, the instruments were unreadable, and the controls about useless. Somehow, I managed to get the nose pointing up more times than down and eventually climbed out of the turbulence. When I got back to Atsugi, the A-4's g meter had registered +9g and −4g, and the fighter grounded for inspection."

Other aircraft flying nearby, but not quite so close to the mountain, also reported severe turbulence.

Ultimately, searchers found the wreckage of the BOAC 707 scattered in a wide path some sixteen kilometers long. As the aircraft had broken up at a considerable height, there was no possibility of survivors, despite much of the fuselage hitting the ground in one piece.

The Investigation

For the investigators, finding out precisely what had happened was difficult because searing heat from burning fuel had seriously damaged the flight data recorder (FDR), which in those days was located in the nose.

The aircraft did not have a cockpit voice recorder (CVR), despite their installation being made mandatory in the United States the year before (1965). In the United Kingdom the pilots' union, like that of their US counterparts, had long opposed the introduction of a "spy in the cockpit," and their installation only became mandatory for UK-registered airliners eight years later.

Thus, with no FDR or CVR, air accident investigators had to try to work out what had happened to the 707 through careful examination of the wreckage and analysis of reports from amateur eyewitnesses, who from the ground could hardly make accurate estimates of the initial height and course of the aircraft. Luckily, the film recovered from a passenger's 8 mm movie camera seemed to answer that question, and it is the basis for the aircraft headings just cited.

As mentioned, it was ascertained that the vertical stabilizer (vertical tail fin) snapped off in a leftward direction and struck the left horizontal stabilizer, causing that to break off too. The ventral stabilizer (an inverted "shark's fin" under the belly beneath the tail) also broke off in a leftward direction, suggesting a powerful leftward gust was responsible rather than overaggressive use of the rudder, as in the case of the Airbus 300 taking off from JFK in 2001.

The passenger's 8 mm movie camera had been filming out of the window when it received a shock sharp enough to skip two frames. Still working, it fell to the floor and showed seats and carpet before stopping. From the footage, investigators estimated that the aircraft had been traveling at a speed of between 320 and 370 knots.

They found some preexisting cracks in the tail area, but tests showed these did not significantly weaken the tail and that some exceptional force must have been at work. Nevertheless, inspections revealed similar cracks in other 707s, and in consequence design changes were made and more frequent inspections ordered.

The loss of two Japan Air Self Defense Force fighters due to severe turbulence near Mount Fuji four years earlier in February 1962 should have been lesson enough, but it was only after this tragic and unnecessary sightseeing accident that the "scenic airway" option was withdrawn.

Wind Shear, Microbursts, and Wake Turbulence (1982 and 1985)

Dangers that catch pilots, and even passengers, unawares

> After a series of wind-shear disasters in the United States, airports most prone to wind shear were belatedly equipped with extremely expensive devices to detect the phenomenon, which have proved highly effective.
>
> Pan American World Airways Flight 759, July 9, 1982
> Delta Flight 191, August 2, 1985
> Delta Air Lines Flight 9570, May 30, 1972

Wind shear occurs where two bodies of air moving in different directions come together. This can result in a dramatic drop in airspeed. Not only can an aircraft find itself going too slowly and stalling, but also the air in the second body may be going downward, thus tending to slam the already vulnerable aircraft into the ground.

One particularly nasty form of wind shear is the microburst. It has a life span of about five to ten minutes and affects an area normally no more than two and a half miles (four kilometers) across. It consists of a small, very intense downdraft that descends to the ground and spreads out in all directions from the point of impact, rather like water from a faucet falling on a flat surface.

Thus, a pilot might take off at the "correct" airspeed into, say, a twenty-knot headwind, with it also pushing him upward and, having gained a modicum of height, suddenly find himself in a thirty-knot tailwind that is also pushing him down faster than the wind that pushed him upward. The fifty-knot drop in airspeed could result in, at worst, a stall, and at least a high sink rate, compounded by the effect of the downward draft, giving the pilot little time to recover, especially if obstacles like trees or perimeter fences lie in his path.

Two incidents in a three-year period made the American traveling public very aware of wind shear and somewhat nervous of flying. Many phoned their congressman, insisting that they do something so that pilots could be forewarned.

Pan American World Airways Flight 759, July 9, 1982
(New Orleans)

ATC had warned of wind shear in all quadrants as the Pan American World Airways Flight 759 prepared for takeoff from New Orleans International Airport. The captain told the first officer to let the speed build up on takeoff and said they would switch off the air-conditioning, so the forward engines would be able to provide more power.

These precautions were to no avail, for after takeoff the aircraft rose to roughly 100 feet (60 meters) and then began to sink. It seemed it might manage to stay in the air, especially as the ground effect would come into play, but at an altitude of some 50 feet (15 meters) it struck some trees 2,376 feet (724 meters) from the end of the runway. Losing further height, it continued, clipping trees and houses, before crashing in a residential area 2,234 feet (681 meters) further on, destroying six houses and substantially damaging five more.

The impact, explosion, and fire that followed resulted in the deaths of all 145 on board and 8 people on the ground, making a final death toll of 153.

The inquiry concluded that the accident was due to microburst-induced wind shear, and that part of the problem would have been the pilot being unaware of what was happening, notably the reversal of wind direction and downward push associated with the microburst phenomenon.

The fact that the total distance from the end of the runway to the crash site was about 4,610 feet (1,405 meters) shows how they might very easily have been able to recover. No doubt the initial strike with the trees, and further clipping of trees and houses, impaired the performance of the aircraft.

This was an example of what can happen when taking off. In an incident three years later, the aircraft was attempting to land.

Delta Flight 191, August 2, 1985 (Dallas/Fort Worth)

There were thunderstorms in the area of the Texas airport as Delta Flight 191, an L1011 jumbo jet with 163 passengers and crew on board, approached Runway 17L (the left of two or even three parallel runways in a 170-degree direction) for landing. There was a rain shaft and scattered lightning coming from a thunderstorm cell in the airliner's final approach path, but the pilots decided the weather was passable and continued the approach.

Some fifteen to thirty seconds after the L1011 entered the weather, however, the rain and lightning intensified, and the airplane was buffeted by a violent series of up-and-down drafts. The headwind increased rapidly to twenty-six knots, and then, just as suddenly, switched to a forty-six-knot tailwind, resulting in an abrupt loss of seventy-two knots of airspeed. The jet was only eight hundred feet above the ground when this happened, leaving the pilots little room to maneuver when the airplane began to lose airspeed and altitude at the same time. Thirty-eight seconds later, Delta Flight 191 crashed into the terrain short of the runway, killing all but twenty-six of those on board.

Following this disaster, improved weather radar was set up at US airports where microburst were frequent, and NASA did research on onboard systems to detect them as notification from the ground can incur fatal delays. They found the most effective system was Doppler radar, now with commercial aircraft around the world equipped with such systems crashes due to microbursts should be something in the past.

Wake Turbulence

One phenomenon, wake turbulence—that is, mini-tornadoes or vortices coming off the wingtips of large aircraft—can endanger following aircraft. Surprisingly, the calmer the weather conditions, the more dangerous these are likely to be, as without turbulence to break them up, they can float for miles.

The worst scenario is generally when a large aircraft heavily laden with fuel and passengers is climbing out after takeoff under high power in clean configuration—that is, with flaps, slats, and undercarriage retracted. Air traffic control uses the word "heavy" in the call signs for large jets as an extra warning.

The amount of turbulence generated does not depend purely on size, with the Boeing 767 being well known for nasty turbulence. Airbus is trying to demonstrate that the wake turbulence generated by its superjumbo A380 is not commensurate with its size and that it should not be penalized by being designated as requiring extra separation from following aircraft.

Delta Air Lines Flight 9570, May 30, 1972 (Greater SW Airport, Fort Worth)

The first instance of wake turbulence from heavies—large jets, such as the 747, DC-10, 767, 777, and A380—causing a following aircraft to crash was in 1972, shortly after the first ones entered service.

Fortunately, the airliner in question was being operated as a training flight with no passengers and only three crew and an FAA inspector on board. A McDonnell Douglas DC-9-14, it was landing at the Greater Southwest International Airport in Fort Worth, Texas, just after a DC-10 had performed a touch-and-go maneuver on the same runway.

As the DC-9 passed over the runway threshold, wake turbulence from one of the DC-10's wingtips caused it to rock and then roll so much that the right wingtip dipped almost ninety degrees and snagged the ground. The aircraft caught fire as it inverted and veered to the right, ending up 2,370 feet beyond the point where it first made contact. Three of those on board were killed by the trauma of the impact and the fourth by the fire.

Air traffic control had warned the pilots they could expect turbulence, but as they had already twice landed behind the DC-10, the inspectors believed the cry wolf syndrome operated, whereby repeated ATC warnings lose weight. The investigators thought it likely that the pilots believed wake turbulence only represented a danger to tiny aircraft and not to ones as large as the DC-9.

Though the death toll was small, it could have been considerable had it been a normal revenue flight with passengers on board. The NTSB investigators studied the question of wake turbulence extensively and recommended the gap between aircraft be lengthened, especially when flying under visual flight rules, where the pilots are making the judgments.

So many factors can affect wake turbulence, and it can have no effect except when they all come together. In this incident, the relatively calm conditions and flat ground prevented the vortexes from breaking up, the slight crosswind component prevented the vortex from spinning off to the side of the runway, and the slight tailwind component kept it there.

Ice Builds Up Behind De-Icing Boots of Turboprop (Chicago, 1994)

Traversing clouds containing supercooled water droplets

> Ice is a major problem in the Northern US, but resultant crashes normally stem from inadequate deicing prior to takeoff. In this case, the aircraft had an inherent design flaw that only revealed itself in flight under very specific conditions.
>
> Eagle Air 4184, October 31, 1994

The ATR was a French-Italian turboprop airliner suitable for short routes, such as the one from Indianapolis to Chicago. The flight was operated by Simmons Airlines for American Eagle. On board were sixty-four passengers and four crew.

The twenty-nine-year-old captain, Orlando Aguiar, had almost 8,000 hours' flight time, of which 1,548 hours were in the ATR. The thirty-year-old first officer, Jeffrey Gagliano, had 5,000 flight hours, of which 3,657 hours were in the ATR. Both were highly regarded. For one of the two flight attendants, it was her first day with American Eagle.

The flight took off from Indianapolis at 14:55, having been held waiting for forty-two minutes for IFR clearance to O'Hare. Because of the short distance, the ATR was already beginning its descent from its cruising height of 16,300 to 10,000 feet at 15:13. Shortly after leveling off, they were told by a trainee female controller under supervision, whom the pilots between themselves referred to as the "the controller chick," to enter a holding pattern in the expectation that they would have to continue in their race-track circuit for some twenty-five minutes, subsequently extended for a further fifteen minutes. Chicago's O'Hare is always very busy, and in bad weather there can be long delays, with international flights given preference and humble turboprops at the back of the queue.

With the airspeed reduced as they made the holding pattern circuits, the nose of the aircraft had pitched up, making it uncomfortable for the passengers and even for the flight attendants going up and down. They therefore extended the flaps slightly to push the nose down, unaware that this would affect the way ice built up on the wings.

Just before the time they had been told they would have to hold expired, they were authorized to descend to 8,000 feet. As the aircraft speeded up, reaching 186 knots, the overspeed warning sounded to tell them they were going too fast for their fifteen-degree flap setting. Not needing them, they retracted them completely rather than reducing speed.

A difficult-to-place sound coming from the airframe, almost as if it is quivering, can be heard on the CVR. An instant later the flight data recorder shows the control column moving sharply rightward and the aircraft tipping to the right. Together the pilots try to right the control column but find that impossible.

Then, just as it seems they are going to plunge to the ground, the aircraft rights itself, with the pilots seeming to be about to regain control, only for it to happen again, this time with no reprieve, and the aircraft plunges to the ground in a field near a tiny Indiana township called

Roselawn, with it beginning to level out, suggesting if the pilots had had two or three thousand feet more height they could have recovered.

All sixty-eight persons on board were killed, and the force of the impact of the partially inverted aircraft was so great that the wreckage consisted of tiny pieces, though it was not damaged by fire, as the fuel had been scattered by the impact. The site was declared a biohazard because of the state of the fragmented bodies.

The Inquiry

Steve Frederick, another pilot working for Eagle Air and a close friend of the copilot of the crashed ATR, started a campaign, distributing leaflets three weeks after the crash saying the aircraft was dangerous, and he even appeared later on a morning TV show to say the same. The airline not only fired him but managed to have his pilot's license revoked, grounding him for seventeen years. Pilots later refused to fly in icy conditions.

The inquiry concluded that the trainee air traffic controller was in no way responsible, and that the pilots, through no fault of their own, by using fifteen-degree flaps to lower the nose exacerbated the tendency for ice to form on top of the wing behind the deicing boots when flying in cloud with supercooled rain droplets.

When they retracted the flaps due to excess speed on the descent, the nose went up, causing the wing with the ice on top not only to stall but create a powerful vortex at the trailing edge, sucking the aileron upward with such force that without "power steering" pilots could not overcome it, making the aircraft uncontrollable.

Looking at the records, investigators found there had been previous cases, including one over the French Alps, where the aileron had behaved in exactly the same way in icy conditions.

The investigators were not happy with the certification process by the French, which was rubber-stamped by the FAA. Admittedly, it was not easy to foresee the way ice would accrue and make the aileron behave in that way. Overall, the ATR incidents and their history should have been investigated much more thoroughly.

Modifications to the aircraft were made.

US Airlines Use ATR Exclusively in South

The FAA subsequently softened an airworthiness directive stopping the ATR being used in icy conditions, but for PR reasons the US airlines from there on used them exclusively in the warmer south.

Moment of Turbulence Results in a Death (off Japan, 1997)

Why passengers should keep seat belts on

> Passengers scoffing at their captain's suggestion that they keep their seat belts on "just in case" do not realize that a smash against the ceiling panels or other solid objects could quickly wipe that know-all look from their faces.
>
> United Airlines Flight 826, December 28, 1997

Most of the passengers on the United Airlines 747-100 that had taken off from Tokyo's Narita Airport for Honolulu at 9:05 p.m. local time were Japanese holidaymakers planning to spend the extended New Year vacation in the warm climes of Hawaii rather than in wintry Japan.

Two hours out of Narita, they were flying above the Pacific en route to Honolulu at the economical cruising height of thirty-one thousand feet. There were 374 passengers and 19 crew members on board, and some people were moving about the cabin. These included cabin crew with their trolleys, as the passengers had just finished dinner.

Nine hundred and twenty-five miles (1,480 kilometers) east of Tokyo, the aircraft encountered some undulation, and the captain turned the seat belt sign on as a precaution. However, it was not accompanied by a chime, or an announcement in either English or Japanese, so passengers probably gave it less attention than they otherwise might.

The captain also radioed Northwest Flight 90, ahead of him, to ask how the ride was, and he was told it was smooth with an occasional ripple of light turbulence at their altitude.

They then encountered some turbulence, followed, about two minutes after the undulation, by severe turbulence. First the aircraft rose, and then it descended so abruptly that heavy food trolleys hit the ceiling, making indentations, before falling back down on people. A purser gripping a counter found himself upside down with his feet in the air.

One Japanese woman hit the ceiling and fell back in such a contorted way that, despite resuscitation efforts by flight attendants and one of the two doctors on board, she died from her injuries.

Japanese TV broadcast a video taken by a passenger showing screaming passengers being thrown about the cabin and debris in the aisles.

A pilot reassured the frightened passengers over the PA, saying, "We have just hit air turbulence and the aircraft descended thirty meters [almost one hundred feet]. There is no danger of a crash."

The drop must have seemed much more than one hundred feet to the terrified passengers. The 747 then turned back to Tokyo's Narita Airport so the injured could receive medical attention. The captain could have landed on Midway but decided Tokyo would be preferable in view of the better medical facilities.

Though 110 out of the 374 passengers were alleged to have been injured, only 10 were kept in hospital. Nine of the 19 crew members were cited as injured, with three of them in a serious condition.

Examination of the flight data recorder showed that at the moment of most severe turbulence the aircraft had experienced a peak acceleration of +1.81 g, pushing the passengers down in their seats, followed by a negative acceleration of –0.82g, lifting them, pushing the aircraft violently down and them upward.

There are an increasing number of cases of passengers being injured by turbulence when not strapped in. We cite this one, as it shows that even where the severe turbulence does not last long and the aircraft does not drop thousands of feet, people can be injured.

Suggestions for passengers
While it may feel slightly uncomfortable—being pushed hard down on your seat or floor—when an aircraft rises suddenly as in this case, passengers are very likely feeling reassured for at least they are going upward and not going to hit the ground.

However, it may presage as in this case a downward drop for which they are not prepared for they have thereto been resisting positive g.

With negative g—the aircraft suddenly dropping—anything not attached, whether it be items or people, will float or hurtle upward. Even if their upward velocity is not great enough for them to make indentations in the ceiling panels, they have to come down again.

Even if the aircraft simply exits the turbulence, they will come down hard, possibly hurting other people, or if it is a person, seriously injuring them.

While turbulence as severe as this with a flight attendant gripping a counter ending up upside down is most unlikely, anyone walking about the aircraft should not only hold on but try and keep their feet anchored in an upset.

Of course, the best place to be when turbulence looks likely is strapped in your seat. In this respect cabin crew are not so fortunate—nine crew members were injured here, three seriously.

Chapter 13
CONTROLLED FLIGHT
INTO TERRAIN (CFIT)

Autopilot Disengages as Pilots Fiddle with Bulb (Everglades, 1972)

No one flying aircraft

> The 1972 crash of an Eastern Airlines TriStar into Florida's Everglades is often cited as a classic case of an aircraft flying into the ground while ostensibly fully under control. That is, there was nothing wrong with the aircraft or its instruments, and the pilots even knew where they were.
>
> Eastern Air Lines Flight 401, December 29, 1972

As the Eastern Airlines Lockheed TriStar with 176 people aboard, and with the captain, first officer, flight engineer, and a company technician on the flight deck, came in to land at Miami, everything was normal until they lowered the landing gear. Instead of three greens, there were only two; the lamp indicating the nose wheel was down and locked had failed to light up.

The crew informed ATC it wanted to abort the landing and investigate the nature of the problem. ATC instructed them to turn off out of the way of other aircraft and proceed northbound at two thousand feet.

With the autopilot set to maintain that height, the two pilots fiddled with the bulb, ultimately trying to remove it from its socket to see whether it had blown.

Meanwhile, the flight engineer, who had been told by the captain to go down to the avionics bay below to look at the wheel via the observation port, came back and said he could not be sure, and went back to look again, accompanied by the company technician.

While the two of them were away in the avionics bay, the chime indicating a deviation of more than 250 feet from the set height sounded just near the seats they had vacated. Had he been in his usual position, the flight engineer would have heard it, but the two pilots wearing headsets evidently did not.

ATC was also getting concerned about their height, which was down to nine hundred feet, but instead of warning them straightforwardly, he politely asked, "How are things coming along out there?"

The Eastern Airlines TriStar captain's reply that they were returning to land suggested they were in control of the situation.

The descending aircraft continued on in the dark over the Everglades swamp, with nothing showing up on the ground to indicate how near it was—rather like the Peruvian aircraft over the sea described later in this chapter.

Turning the aircraft southward, the first officer noticed the lack of height even though his autopilot light was on. First officer:

We did something to the altitude!

Captain:

What? . . . We're still at two thousand . . . right?

Hey . . . what's happening here?

There was a bleep from the radio altimeters, indicating the proximity of the ground, followed by the sound of the left wing hitting the ground.

The ground proximity warning would certainly have sounded earlier had they unfortunately not been in a left banking turn with the bottom of the aircraft facing sideways rather than straight down.

The left landing gear struck next, after which the aircraft began to break up, with wreckage spread over a swath of flat marshland 1,500 feet long.

The Rescue

It took rescuers thirty minutes to reach the scene in helicopters and airboats (shallow-draft flat-bottom boats with a fan at the back that can skim over the swamp and reeds).

Only two sections of the aircraft were intact—the tail and a section of the cabin. The rest was in pieces.

It is remarkable that 77 out of the 176 persons on board survived. The death toll was 99. The two pilots and the flight engineer were among the fatalities, though the company technician in the jump seat, who had absented himself from the flight deck and was still in the avionics bay to try to check visually from there whether the front wheel was down, did survive.

The Investigation

The investigators attributed the disaster to pilot error.

They said, "It seems that in turning around to tell the flight engineer to go down to the avionics bay, the captain must have exerted a strong force on the control column equivalent to fifteen pounds, thus disengaging the autopilot on his side. Unfortunately, the autopilot on the first officer's side was mistakenly set to only disengage if the applied force exceeded some twenty pounds, compared with rather less on the captain's side. As a result, the light on the first officer's side would have stayed on, giving him the impression that the autopilot was maintaining them at two thousand feet."

"The Ghost of Flight 401"

John Grant Fuller, a non-fiction writer with particular interest in extra-terrestrial events, wrote a book called *The Ghost of Flight 401* based on this crash, describing how Eastern Air Lines crews on Lockheed L-1011s with replacement parts recovered from the one that crashed convincingly reported seeing the ghosts of the pilots and flight engineer who died.

In 1978 it was turned into a popular TV movie with the same name. The airline thought of suing but feared that would engender even more publicity, with people giving the "rubbish" some credence. Instead they opted to remove all the cannibalized parts.

Preprogrammed to Hit Mount Erebus (Antarctica, 1979)

A question of command responsibility?

> This accident, in which a DC-10 full of sightseers flew into a mountain at the South Pole, took place at a time when the advantage of using computers to manage the flight was beginning to be exploited.
>
> Air New Zealand Flight 901, November 28, 1979

Staff at Air New Zealand's Flight Operations Division had a sinking feeling of culpability in the pit of their stomachs on learning their sightseeing DC-10 had flown straight into a mountain at the South Pole, for that was precisely what they had programmed it to do!

Without informing the pilots, they had made a correction to the final waypoint the night before, moving it from the end of McMurdo Sound, where the track to it passed over water, to a point behind Mount Erebus, where the track would pass right over the 12,450-foot-high mountain. The airline's chief executive then compounded the scandal by appropriating and shredding documents to try to cover up their mistake.

The scandalous aspect that made the affair a cause célèbre in normally uneventful New Zealand is not why this disaster is of particular interest here. Rather, it is because it highlights three common elements essential for preventing air accidents:

1. Command responsibility

2. Cockpit resource management (CRM)

3. Consideration of all possibilities when something odd happens and taking conservative action if any doubt remains.

"Command responsibility" is the tenet that the captain of a ship or aircraft has the ultimate responsibility for ensuring his passengers' and vessel's safety, whatever the pressures put on him by management or circumstances.

There are no excuses. It represents responsibility to a higher God—professionalism in the best sense of the word. Something the captain of the Titanic apparently did not demonstrate.

CRM is the concept that the crew works as a team, with even the lesser players able to contribute. In this case, that person's contribution came twenty-six seconds before the impact, with a flight engineer registering his increasing disquiet by saying, "I don't like this!"

In fact, both flight engineers had been getting increasingly concerned.

"Consideration of all possibilities" relates to the fact that the crew assumed they could not receive the VHF radio transmissions from the US base for some technical reason without thinking that it could be because high land, possibly a mountain, blocked their path.

The Disaster

As in the case of the BOAC sightseeing disaster near Japan's Mount Fuji and the Airbus crash at the Habsheim Air Show, jaunts with sightseeing passengers on board are inherently more dangerous than serious commercial flights, as they tend to generate an easygoing attitude and involve unfamiliar routes and circumstances.

Air New Zealand's sightseeing trips to the South Pole were no exception. However, involving a six-thousand-nautical-mile flight lasting up to twelve hours, they represented a major operation. Weather conditions permitting, the aircraft would descend to two thousand feet near the Pole for a better view. This low-level flying would consume fuel at a high rate, and even with a virtually full load of fuel at takeoff, the DC-10 would be operating without much margin for playing around before the long return leg home.

Before the introduction of GPS, navigation on long routes over water with no radio beacons depended upon inertial navigation systems (INS), which were and are also used for guiding intercontinental ballistic missiles (ICBMs).

The idea behind INS is quite simple.

1. A combination of gyroscopes measures changes of direction.
2. Sensors attached to inertial weights detect acceleration and deceleration.
3. A computer integrates the two to calculate the position.

The system is in triplicate, allowing the computer to ascertain if one has failed, as it will be the odd man out. As with ballistic missiles, users can program the desired route into the system so the aircraft flies to the destination automatically.

In airline use, the system works very well provided the pilots put in the correct coordinates. This has perhaps not always been the case (see Korean Airlines 747 Shot Down over Russia).

The INS system is a form of dead reckoning, so, unlike the GPS system, which is based on satellites, accuracy decreases with time and distance. Some versions are referred to as AINS (area INS) in that they are considered accurate over a specific area.

These Air New Zealand trips to Antarctica were popular with airline staff, and in consequence rather than choosing pilots with experience of polar flying, the treat was ill advisedly shared out as a perk. The captain chosen that time was forty-five-year-old Captain Collins. He had eleven thousand hours' flying experience, three thousand of them on the DC-10. A qualified navigator, he was regarded as a very capable pilot who exercised good judgment, but he lacked experience of flying in Arctic conditions.

The rest of the flight crew consisted of two first officers, Cassin and Lucas, and two flight engineers, Brooks, forty-four, and Moloney, forty-nine. Brooks had been on one previous flight to the Antarctic, while Maloney had the most airline experience.

As usual on these trips, a celebrity was included, his role being to give a commentary to the passengers on approaching the South Pole. This time it was Peter Mulgrew, a well-known New Zealand adventurer, who had walked from McMurdo (the DC-10's first objective) to the South Pole on an expedition led by Sir Edmund Hillary, famed for climbing Mount Everest.

On board the DC-10 were 237 passengers. Though most were New Zealanders, people of other nationalities, including 24 Japanese and 23 Americans, were present. There was also a sizable cabin crew to indulge them. In all, 257 excited souls were departing from Auckland that November 28, 1979 morning, never to return.

McMurdo is US exploration base 2,384 miles from Auckland. With a thousand visitors in summer and two hundred or so residents in winter, it had long been the main point of entry for those venturing into Antarctica. Late November would be summer, with daylight lasting twenty-four hours a day. Nearby is the much smaller New Zealand Scott base.

McMurdo has an ice runway able to take certain types of aircraft—weather conditions permitting. There was no question of the DC-10 touching down there; they only wanted to avail themselves of the base's radar facilities so they could be safely talked down to get a better view.

Next to McMurdo was Ross Island, with various peaks, the highest being Mount Erebus (12,450 feet) and Mount Terror (10,700 feet), named after the two ships, under the command of Englishman Captain Ross, that came to the area in 1841, and, fearful of being iced in, did not attempt to make land.

Mount Erebus is actually an active volcano. In satellite photos the red-hot magma at the peak looks scary against the snowy whiteness of the surrounding slopes. Despite appearances, Ross Island is a true island, being joined to mainland Antarctica only by a vast ice shelf.

The planned outward route from Auckland would take the DC-10 out over the sea, over New Zealand's South Island and on to the Antarctic. They would pass over a number of waypoints, including a couple of tiny islands, which would enable them to confirm their position and hence the accuracy of their INS navigation system. Interestingly, the nearer they got to the South Pole, the greater the discrepancy between their true heading and magnetic heading would become, attaining as much as 160 degrees at McMurdo. Indeed, at McMurdo anyone on the ground would find the compass needle pointing downward!

The last waypoint before McMurdo was Cape Hallet. According to the unrevised map the pilots had worked on prior to the trip, the McMurdo waypoint was on low-lying ground, with just sea in between the two waypoints. The nearest they would come to Mount Erebus should have been twenty to twenty-five nautical miles, and with relatively little distance covered after passing over Cape Hallet, there could hardly be an INS error of that magnitude.

In fact, it was a pity the INS was performing so well. With the McMurdo waypoint reprogrammed to be two degrees ten seconds of longitude farther east, the direct track to it from Cape Hallet passed not over the sea but right over the mountain!

While still some way off McMurdo, the DC-10 was able to contact the base on VHF, but as the base replied on HF, both parties opted for HF, as that is less affected by distance and obstacles. In addition, being so far from anywhere, there would not be the usual interference from other transmissions.

McMurdo informed them that there was still low overcast at two thousand feet with some snow, but that visibility remained about forty miles. The DC-10 requested permission to descend to Flight Level 160 (sixteen thousand feet) but was only authorized to descend to Flight Level 180, eighteen thousand feet.

McMurdo then said: "Within range of forty miles of McMurdo we have radar that will, if you desire, let you down to 1,500 feet on radar vectors. Over."

This pleased the DC-10 captain and first officer, who were getting worried their trip would be a washout. Thinking that the visibility was good enough for them to make a descent, perhaps performing an orbit (circle) to keep out of the cloud ahead, the captain said, "Well, actually it's clear out here if we get down."

To which the flight engineer said, "It's not clear on the right-hand side here."

The first officer agreed, saying, "No." Despite the comment from the flight engineer, the first officer called McMurdo at the captain's request, saying: "We'd like further descent and we could orbit in our present position, which is approximately forty-three miles north, descending in VMC"

VMC meant visual meteorological conditions and implied they could see the ground and around them clearly.

McMurdo gave permission and asked to be kept informed of their height, and the DC-10 acknowledged and confirmed they were vacating Flight Level 180.

With only three miles to go before they should be on the McMurdo radar, it is surprising that the captain should have opted to go to the trouble of circling to descend in a clear part of sky where visibility on the right was not so clear. Was he trying to give his passengers a better view?

For a moment, the VHF radio seemed to be working. They then reverted to HF without considering that the inability to communicate by line-of-sight VHF could be because they were in the wrong location. They then called McMurdo on HF:

901 . . . still negative contact on VHF. We are VMC and we'd like to let down on a grid of one eight zero and proceed visually to McMurdo.

McMurdo replied:

New Zealand 901 maintain VMC. Keep us advised of your altitude as you approach McMurdo . . .

Conversing in the cockpit, the captain said he had VMC "This way," and that he was "Go[ing?]." At the same moment, Mulgrew, the guide, frustrated at not being able to earn his keep, was saying to the others in the cockpit, "Ah well, you can't talk if you can't see anything . . . Here you go. There's some land ahead."

The first officer informed McMurdo that they were descending from six thousand feet to two thousand and that they were VMC. The captain said he had heard there was clear weather at a place called Wright Valley and seemed to be asking Mulgrew whether he could get them there. He thought he could. Perhaps getting worried, the flight engineer said, "Where's Erebus in relation to us at the moment?"

After saying, "Left, about twenty or twenty-five miles," and some discussion, Mulgrew admitted he did not really know. They then finally all agreed that conditions did not look good. The flight engineer, expressing his concern more strongly, exclaimed, "I don't like this!"

The captain, presumably relying on the INS, said they were twenty-nine nautical miles north and that they would have to climb out of it.

The first officer declared, "You're clear to turn right. There's no high ground if you do a one-eighty."

Thereupon the GPWS (ground proximity warning system), operating with a six-second delay to prevent spurious warnings, went:

Whoop! Whoop! Pull up! Whoop! Whoop!

The first officer announced they were at "five hundred feet."

GPWS:

Pull up!

The first officer announced, "Four hundred feet."

GPWS:

Whoop! Whoop! Pull up! Whoop! Whoop! Pull up!

Politely, the captain asked for go-around power; he did not push the throttles through the gates (to get maximum power at the sacrifice of engine life), so he could not have seen anything to indicate a mountain was ahead.

The last words on the CVR tape were from the GPWS:

Whoop! Whoop! Pull—

Crash into the Mountain

Five minutes later the McMurdo controller, wanting to find out why they were taking so long to confirm their descent to 2,000 feet, called them both on VHF and HF and repeatedly thereafter, to no avail. It was not until the next day and eleven hours later that a US Navy Hercules searching the northern part of Ross Island reported finding the wreckage and the absence of survivors.

The DFDR (digital flight data recorder) showed the aircraft had made two descending orbits either side of its track as it descended and leveled out at 1,500 feet.

Continuing on at that height, it had impacted the thirteen-degree-upward slope of Mount Erebus at 240 knots, with a nose-up angle of ten degrees as the pilots attempted their last-minute go-around.

With the landing gear up and only a thin layer of powdery snow covering the hard layer of ice coating the slope, there was nothing to cushion the shock, and the aircraft skidded up the slope for a distance of some 550 meters, breaking up as it went. Traces of fire showed on the ice.

Unlike crashes where there is some warning of impending disaster, passengers in CFIT disasters are not usually wearing seat belts, and certainly not in the brace position. In this case, many were thrown clear as the aircraft broke up. A large number of the bodies were surprisingly intact, but postmortems showed they died from the initial impact.

Had the pilots seen the slope ahead and raised the nose earlier and more sharply, the aircraft might have been climbing and losing speed, making the shock of the impact with the incline much less severe, and raising the possibility that there might have been survivors. However, one wonders, as with the Japan Airlines crash, how many traumatized survivors could last a whole night in the cold.

So great was the shock to that small nation, and so great was the scandal, that two inquiries were launched:

1. The usual New Zealand Office of Air Accidents inquiry, led by Chief Inspector Chippendale.
2. A special Royal Commission of Inquiry, under the royal commissioner, Mr. Justice P. T. Mahon, who overturned their findings.

The former attributed the accident to:

> The decision of the captain to continue the flight at low level toward an area of poor surface and horizon definition when the crew were not certain of their position, and their subsequent inability to detect the rising terrain that intercepted the aircraft's flight path.

(2) The royal commissioner's summation was very different:

> "In my opinion the single dominant and effective cause of the disaster was the mistake made by those airline officials who programmed the aircraft to fly directly at Mount Erebus and omitted to tell the aircrew. That mistake is directly attributable not so much to the persons who made it, but to the incompetent administrative airline procedures, which made the mistake possible.

> Neither Captain Collins nor the flight engineers made any error which contributed to the disaster and were not responsible for its occurrence."

Whiteout Plus Whole Series of Mistakes

The fact that aviation experts and legal experts could come to such different conclusions is interesting. In the present author's view, the truth lies somewhere between these two extremes and is tipped against the pilots.

The airline's mistake in not informing the pilots of the revision they had made is blatant, and it is more than understandable that the Royal Commission was revolted at the way the chief executive attempted to cover it up. The commission was also of course dismayed that the flag carrier, albeit of a tiny country, was run close to the CEO's chest like a private fiefdom. These sentiments, rather than technical matters, were bound to influence "professionals used to working in the judicial domain."

The actual key to the accident was a phenomenon called "whiteout," well known to pilots operating in areas with snow and mountains, whereby the snowy slopes merge with the clouds, giving the impression there is just thin cloud in the distance.

The horizon disappears. A pilot without experience of the phenomenon or proper training in Arctic flying would be left with the impression it is safe to fly visually (VMC), as he believes he can see in the immediate vicinity. Under visual flight rules, this gave the pilots the regulatory justification for descending, as Captain Gordon Vette, author of Impact Erebus, pointed out at the tribunal.

If the key to the disaster was whiteout, then the airline should be faulted for treating the Antarctic flights as perks to be shared around and not choosing pilots with Antarctic experience.

Failing that, briefing on whiteout and Arctic flying should have been better. On the other hand, it is difficult to understand why the pilots did not become concerned not only by their inability to communicate with McMurdo by VHF but also by their failure to lock on to either of the (VHF) radio beacons there. The two flight engineers were getting increasingly worried, and finally the captain agreed they should go around, but too late.

One can only conclude that the wish to please the passengers got the better of the captain, with lack of knowledge of how deceptive a whiteout can be as a mitigating factor.

The fact that he performed two orbits to remain under VMC proves he wanted to stick to regulations and not fly blindly into cloud. As he was just three miles from the forty-miles-out line, from where the base radar would have been able to talk him down, he must have been pretty sure of the weather conditions.

When they realized they could not see where they were, they should have acted immediately. Possibly the presence of the tour guide in the cockpit, and his interceding to give his opinion as to where they might be, slowed decision-making.

The airline's monumental blunder was just one factor in an accident that would not have happened had due weight been given to command responsibility, cockpit resource management (CRM), and the need to explore all possibilities when something (in this case the VHF radio and radio beacons) is not working—a dramatic and sorry lesson for everyone.

Air Inter Airbus A320 Plows into Mountain (Sainte-Odile, 1992)
No ground proximity warning system (GPWS)

> Facing increasing competition from high-speed trains, France's domestic airline, Air Inter, with many short-distance flights, was shortening flight times, descending unusually quickly on landing, and likely to trigger GPWS.
>
> Air Inter Flight 148, January 20, 1992

Another notable feature of this incident was that two senior captains were flying the aircraft. From a cockpit resources management (CRM) point of view, that is undesirable, as the normal senior-versus-junior relationship breaks down, and corners are sometimes cut. Despite their rank, the Air Inter captains making up the duo had little experience of flying the A320—only 160 and 60 hours respectively.

Air Inter was France's major domestic airline until it merged with Air France on April 1, 1997. Unlike British European Airways, which was the poor relation when it merged with long-haul BOAC to form British Airways, the working conditions at Air Inter were even more favorable than at Air France, for Air Inter had been carrying businesspeople and the rich on protected routes.

The flight that led to this A320 disaster was one such flight, a short cross-country hop from France's second city, Lyon, to Strasbourg with ninety passengers, four cabin crew, and two pilots. It was winter, it was dark, and although ground visibility was six miles (ten kilometers), there were clouds above 600 feet, with the tops some 1,500 feet higher. The Vosges Mountains were nearby.

The captain flying the aircraft had approval from the tower to make a straight-in VOR DME approach and landing. Finding he was too high and going too fast, he asked the controller to be allowed to continue as if landing but overfly the runway, and on reaching the opposite outer marker, double back downwind using the ILS until able to turn back again to make a visual approach to the runway.

He was informed that if he did this, he would probably be kept in a holding pattern until the three aircraft waiting to depart had done so. He decided to land as originally intended, using the VOR DME approach.

With the approval of the approach controller, who told him to maintain 5,000 feet and gave him the required vectors that should have brought him in the vicinity of Andlau and well-positioned for a run straight to the airport over relatively low ground, the captain executed the almost 360-degree circuit.

Although there were mountains in the vicinity, and even higher peaks northwest of Andlau, flying at a height of 5,000 feet and with no need to descend steeply, there should have been an ample safety margin, even if off course. According to the radar, after being at 5,000 feet for a minute, the aircraft descended 2,700 feet in the next minute, which was a ridiculous rate of descent in the circumstances.

With no warning, they hit one of Mount La Bloss's ridges at the 2,625-foot (800-meter) level. Had they been just a little higher or made a slightly wider turn to actually pass over Andlau, they would not have hit the ground. Of course, they should have been very much higher at that point.

At the time of impact, the aircraft was, unbelievably, descending at an angle of twelve degrees and banking at about eighteen degrees to the left. It cut a swath through the trees on the pine-tree-covered slope and caught fire. Eight passengers and a cabin attendant survived. Had the emergency locator beacons been capable of withstanding the fire, another six passengers could have been saved. As it was, survivors had to huddle near a fire at the tail to keep warm, soon joined by some journalists who had found rescue vehicles waiting on a road lower down—the journalists had simply gone up and followed the smell of fuel. On finding the wreckage they had phoned the rescue services, who still did not come.

The cockpit voice recorder (CVR) was recovered intact, while the flight data recorder (FDR), located only a few inches away, was too damaged to provide any useful information, despite being designed to withstand fires of 1,100°C for thirty minutes. One reason for the damage was that the FDR had been left untouched lying for a long time in the vicinity of flames. This was because accusations that the French investigators and authorities had tampered with the recorders in an earlier Air France Airbus A320 crash at an airshow in 1988 meant that only someone from the judiciary could take them.

However, the quick access recorder (QAR) used for maintenance and not designed to resist fire but situated in the nose was relatively undamaged and provided useful data though not nearly as much as the main one would have.

It took the investigators six hundred and seventy-six days to issue their final report. They could not understand why the aircraft had descended so rapidly just immediately prior to the impact. They had noticed a coincidence that the aircraft should have had a glide slope of -3.3 degrees but that the pilot must have entered it into the flight control unit (FCU) as a vertical descent of – 3,300 feet a minute, probably because it was set in the "Heading/Vertical Speed" mode instead of in the "Track/Flight Path" mode.

It was a mistake easily made and not easily noticed because the designers of the instrument panel only showed the figure entered into the FCU to two decimal places, thus -3,300 feet displayed as -33, which when quickly scanned visually could be taken for -3.3. However, when this was tried in the simulator, the aircraft still missed the mountain by a fair margin. Nonplussed, the investigators went to the manufacturer, Airbus, to see if they could explain why the aircraft had descended even faster, learned that to cope with emergency situations the descent is enhanced.

The pilots received no warning that they were sinking at an alarming rate or about to hit the ground, because there was no ground proximity warning system (GPWS).

The French weekly magazine *Le Point* is said to have questioned Air Inter on this point and to have been told that Air Inter's pilots only flew in France and knew the terrain so well they did not need GPWS.

Apparently, only five weeks before the crash, M. Frantzen, director of the aeronautical training and technical control service, enjoined Air Inter by letter to reconnect these alarm systems but was sent packing. The sophisticated GPWS that has prevented many crashes would not only have warned the pilots of the proximity of the terrain but also of the abnormally high sink rate, an alert that the pilots in the Indian Airlines disaster described above ignored.

In the absence of FDR evidence, due to heat damage to the tape, attributing the cause of the crash to the easy confusion over the input mode seems quite plausible, but some people are not convinced the whole truth has been revealed.

On a website called EuroCockpit, there is a piece on the affair saying that instead of VOR Bendix + DME TRT, as used by Air France, Air Inter had a different type of system (VOR + DME-Collins). It also claims that Lufthansa, among others, had forbidden the use of that system for VOR DME approaches six months before the crash, and that Air Inter did likewise after the crash and an incident at Bordeaux.

According to EuroCockpit, it was a problem of hurried certification, and it says it is rumored that the woman elevated to head the Inspection Générale de l'Aviation Civile was previously responsible for VOR DME certification. Also, it is claimed that the records of receiving reports sent by Air Inter staff to Airbus and the BEA regarding problems with the Collins version have disappeared without trace, even though there are records of them being sent.

Allegedly, the CVR tape for the St Odile crash showed the pilots were somewhat casual, perhaps because it was two captains together. Macarthur Job suggested the nature of Air Inter's routes, with many automatic landings in bad weather, may have made them depend too much on the computers in controlling height.

That said, the disarming of the GPWS by Air Inter seems unforgivable. One reason for so many false alerts was to compete with France's ultrafast new trains Air Inter was bringing its flights into land faster than the norm with rapid descent rates. For a long time, pilots blocked the introduction of the TCAS collision alert system on similar grounds and said that it just meant an extra thing to think about.

This accident is also notable for the continuing litigation involved, with proceedings taking place even in 2009, some seventeen years later! The Echo Association, founded by the victims' families, commented on how one court would come to one conclusion only for it to be reversed another.

One must have some sympathy for the victims' families seeking justice. Aviation in France is a very close-knit incestuous community.

757 Captain Selects Wrong Beacon, Loses Way (Cali, 1995)

Air brakes prevent pilots extricating themselves

> How could a state-of-the-art airliner with a sophisticated, almost automatic navigation system go off course?
>
> American Airlines Flight 965, December 20, 1995

So much of modern airliner piloting is routine. On regularly scheduled flights the dispatchers, or the pilots, load a previously prepared flight plan into the flight management system with all the waypoints and so on. It prevents errors and, of course, saves considerable time. However, it means pilots, not having to enter the waypoints themselves, do not see where the designation for a waypoint beacon might be confusing.

American Airlines Flight 965 to Cali, Colombia, from Miami had taken off two hours late because of the delayed arrival of connecting passengers from the US's northeast, hit by a storm, and a very long wait before entering the runway due to congestion.

The experienced pilots of the Boeing 757, with 163 passengers and 8 crew, were therefore keen to make up time.

The fifty-seven-year-old captain had flown to Cali dozens of times, the last time only six days earlier, but this was the thirty-seven-year-old copilot's first trip there, which is one reason that he might have deferred to the captain's judgment more than usual.

Flying over Cuban airspace, they began their approach into Cali, situated on a plain at the end of a long valley straddled by high mountains, some of which are almost fourteen thousand feet high, after only about three hours.

Unlike most airports, where the approach controller follows incoming aircraft on his or her radar, Cali could not do so, because FARC antigovernment fighters had blown up the installation. Instead, the controller had to rely on the pilots reporting their positions as they passed over various beacons, and a key part of this was a radio beacon far up the valley called Tuluá.

The captain told the controller his distance-measuring equipment (DME) showed they were sixty-three nautical miles from Cali, whereupon, while telling him to report on passing Tuluá, the controller confirmed he was "cleared directly" to Cali. For some reason, the captain thought this meant he could forget about Tuluá, although in his read back he mechanically ended with "report Tuluá." He reset the flight management system to take them directly to Cali, in the process erasing all the waypoints in between, including Tuluá.

Cali Airport only had one runway, roughly aligned with the valley, and with the prevailing wind usually coming from the valley, aircraft would normally skirt the airport and land from the opposite direction. This was what was programmed into the flight management system, meaning the pilots could land almost automatically with no hassle. However, noticing that the wind had dropped, the controller gave them the option of a straight-in landing.

This appealed to the captain, aware that the delay in departing from Miami meant the cabin attendants might not have sufficient rest time, and the return flight the following morning would be delayed. The pilots were happy to accept the offer, although it would require some feverish activity, losing height, and consulting paper charts to note waypoints and frequencies. They did not have time to do this in a calm and collected way and keep a proper eye on what the aircraft was doing.

The first officer deployed the air brakes, which are rectangular panels on top of the wings that flip up and not only slow it but push it downward without putting the nose down and making the passengers uncomfortable. This made the aircraft descend more rapidly.

Fumbling with the chart, they saw they must enter a waypoint called Rozo into the system. Meanwhile, the controller repeatedly asked them to confirm when passing Tuluá, but they had no idea where it was, having erased it from their computer and with no time to find a way to find it.

The captain asked the controller if it was okay to go to Rozo and was told what to do after that, with the controller again asking him to report passing Tuluá.

Realizing they must anyway have already passed it, the captain entered Rozo into the system by pressing "R" on the panel. Ten options came up, none of which were Rozo.

But as the nearest one is usually shown first, and that could in the captain's mind only be Rozo, the captain hastily and fatally confirmed that, without getting his copilot to verify.

If the copilot had verified, he would have seen the system showing a track taking them more than ninety degrees to the left, which was obviously wrong.

The flight management system duly executed the captain's instruction and, with the aircraft descending, gently but surely, turned it left through an angle of some 120 degrees so it passed over the mountains and headed for the Romeo beacon, at Bogota Airport, 172 miles (300 kilometers) away.

There is a rule that, apart from when cruising, one pilot should constantly watch what the aircraft is doing, but in this case, they were both too busy concentrating on the charts and did not notice the aircraft turning. After a minute or so, they began to realize they were obviously heading for the wrong place. For a moment, they considered inputting Tuluá, but the captain then decided they should head straight for Cali, which they did know. What they did not realize was that while still high they had passed over the mountains into the next, almost parallel valley.

The controller with no radar called them to ascertain their height, which they confirmed was nine thousand feet.

Heading for the Cali CLO beacon took them back over the high mountain ridge separating the valleys.

With them lower than before, the ground proximity warning system (GPWS) alerted them to terrain. Unsure of how high it was, they applied full power to climb, but still the warning system kept sounding, and as they got closer it said, "Pull up! Pull up!"

Had they not left the air brakes deployed, the powerful Boeing 757 would almost certainly have gained enough height to surmount the ridge, but as it was it crashed into the trees right at the top, with part of the aircraft sliding over.

The crash site was six miles south of Tuluá VOR and twenty-eight miles north of the runway. As the controller had no operating radar, the location of the crash was not immediately obvious, and rescuers did not reach it until the following morning to look for survivors. They found five, one of whom died later in hospital of internal injuries.

The Inquiry
Many items from the wreckage were spirited away by thieves arriving by military helicopter and ended up on the black market in the US, with American Airlines publishing a list with the part numbers to try and dissuade purchasers. Fortunately, the cockpit voice recorder and flight data recorder were recovered intact, as was the flight management system, which was not much use, since its memory did not at the time retain deleted settings.

The inquiry was carried out very professionally by the Bolivians with the help of the NTSB and found amongst other things that:

1. The flight crew had insufficient time to prepare for the approach to Runway 19 before beginning the approach.

2. The flight crew failed to discontinue the approach despite their confusion regarding elements of the approach and numerous cues indicating the inadvisability of continuing.

3. Many important differences existed between the display of identical navigation data on approach charts and on FMS-generated displays, despite the fact that the same supplier provided American Airlines with the navigational data.

4. The AA965 flight crew was not informed or aware of the fact that the "R" identifier that appeared on the approach chart (Rozo) did not correspond to the "R" identifier (Romeo) that they entered and executed as an FMS command.

5. One of the AA965 pilots selected a direct course to the Romeo NDB, believing that it was the Rozo NDB and, upon executing the selection in the FMS, permitted a turn of the airplane toward Romeo without having verified that it was the correct selection and without having first obtained approval of the other pilot, contrary to AA's procedures.

6. The incorrect FMS entry led to the airplane departing the inbound course to Cali and turning it toward Bogota. The subsequent turn to intercept the extended centerline of the runway led to the turn toward high terrain.

7. The descent was continuous from FL 230 until the crash.

8. Neither pilot recognized that the speed brakes were extended during the GPWS escape maneuver due to the lack of clues available to alert them about the extended condition.
9. Considering the remote, mountainous terrain, the search and rescue response was timely and effective.
10. Although five passengers initially survived, this was considered a nonsurvivable accident due to the destruction of the cabin.
11. The Cali approach controller followed applicable ICAO and Colombian air traffic control rules and did not contribute to the cause of the accident.
12. AA training policies did not include provision for keeping pilots' flight training records, which indicated any details of pilot performance.

Elsewhere in this book we have regretted how difficult it is to discover the finer reservations an airline might have had regarding a pilot's performance, other than that he or she possibly after failing finally passed the required tests during training and route checking.

Some airlines may avoid keeping discoverable records lest the information be used against them in litigation.

Aftermath
American Airlines were sued, and though they were obliged to pay in a number of cases, they in turn sued Jeppesen and Honeywell, who made the navigation computer database and did not include the coordinates of Rozo under the identifier "R."

The jury trial in Miami found that Jeppesen was 30 percent at fault for the crash, Honeywell was 10 percent at fault, and American Airlines 60 percent.

Having unsophisticated juries decide these complex situations is questionable. One only has to remember the SilkAir "suicide" crash, where the jury held Parker Hannifin responsible without being allowed to see the contrary NTSB's findings.

757 Hits Sea as ATC Confirms Altitude as 9,700 Feet (Lima, 1996)

"Two-dollar-per-hour aircraft polisher" brings down jet

> When the worried pilots asked ATC to confirm their altitude, the controller was unwittingly only sending back the erroneous one shown on their altimeter.
>
> Aeroperú Flight 603, October 2, 1996

For the Aeroperú pilots, the flight had been a nightmare from the moment they lifted off on departure from Lima. The incorrect data that was making the altimeter and airspeed indicator give erroneous readings was making the aircraft's computers believe the aircraft was flying outside the normal envelope. In consequence, it was issuing a barrage of warnings and setting off a tirade off aural alarms.

Pilots are trained to react to alarms, and when these come in rapid succession for no rhyme or reason and seem unconnected, one can imagine the crew's confusion. For instance, reducing engine power and deploying the air brakes in response to an overspeed alert did not seem to have any effect—at least according to the airspeed indicator, which was not functioning properly. Sometimes they would get a stick shake, indicating they were about to stall because of inadequate airspeed while being simultaneously warned they were going too fast.

Perhaps out of habit or because they were too busy coping with the crises and different alarms, or even regressing mentally, the Aeroperú pilots failed to note that, in contrast to the barometric altimeter, the radio altimeter showed changes in height corresponding with what they would expect, according to their engine settings and pitch—climbing, level, or descending.

With the incessant warnings and the need to cope with them, it is understandable that the pilots had little time to think. Hardly had they tried to deal with one when another sounded, and audio alarms are particularly stressful.

To give some idea of the confusion, here is part of the CVR (translated from Spanish), beginning about seven minutes before they struck the water. Times in parentheses are elapsed time in minutes and seconds from takeoff (00:00).

22:42 First officer to ATC:

We have terrain alarm; we have terrain alarm!

22:46 Lima ATC:

Roger, according to the monitor. . . it indicates Flight Level 120 [12,000 feet] over the sea, heading northwest course of three hundred.

22:55 First officer to ATC:

We have terrain alarm and we are supposed to be at 10,000 feet?

23:00 Lima ATC:

According to monitor you have one, zero, five [10,500 feet].

23:03 Mechanical voice alert:

Wind shear! Wind shear! Wind shear!

23:06 First officer to ATC:

We have all computers crazy here . . .

23:07 Mechanical voice alert:
Too low, terrain!

23:07 Captain:
Shit, we have everything!

23:14 Mechanical voice alert:
Wind shear! Wind shear! Wind shear!

23:17 Captain:
Shit, what the hell have these assholes [maintenance] done?

23:47 First officer to ATC:
We don't have . . . We have, like, 370 knots. Are we descending now?

23:56 Lima ATC:
It shows the same speed . . . you have approximately 200 speed.

23:56 First officer to ATC:
Speed of 200?

23:58 Lima ATC:
Speed of 220 over the ground, speed reducing slightly.

24:05 Captain:
Shit! We will stall now . . .

24:07 Mechanical voice alert:
Sink rate! Sink rate! Sink rate!
Sink rate!

They managed to avoid stalling and climbed, with the barometric altimeters showing over 9,000 feet. They thought they had leveled out at Flight Level 100 (10,000 feet), a nice, safe altitude.

However, the flight data recorder (FDR) later showed that the radio altimeter indicated they had only climbed to 2,400 feet, then re-descended to 1,300 feet, and had finally gone no higher than 4,000 feet.

Meanwhile, by noting their different locations with his civilian radar, which could independently determine distance and direction (but not true height, which depended on that reported from the aircraft by the transponder), the air traffic controller had calculated their groundspeed to be 200 knots, when the pilots' instruments were showing their airspeed to be 370 knots. To have a difference of that magnitude between groundspeed and airspeed would require a wind over 200 mph. The first officer was surprised, but for some reason it did not immediately make him doubt the overspeed warnings. Perhaps his reaction to them was an understandable automatic reaction to alarms in general.

Unsure of their height, they had gone out over the sea to play it safe. Had they remained over land, they might very well have seen some lights that would have shown how extremely low they were, and because of the presence of hills and mountains would have given more weight to the accurate readings shown by their radio altimeter.

The controller had informed them that a Boeing 707 taking off from Lima was coming to assist them and would guide them in. Without waiting, they thought that already being relatively near the airport it would be a good idea to try to lock onto the airport's instrument landing system (ILS) glide path, which in normal circumstances would have enabled them to descend safely without relying on their instruments. However, unbeknown to them, they were far too low to pick up the beam.

Unfortunately for the occupants of the Aeroperú 757, civil aviation radar, which is not intended for tracking an enemy trying to sneak in, relies on the transponder in the aircraft to give it its altitude and ID. So, when the Aeroperú crew asked ATC to confirm their height, ATC was only repeating what the barometric altimeters in the aircraft showed.

Some suggest that this fact was overlooked because all were convinced it was a computer problem. The airline did try to contact the pilots and find out what was happening, but staff there were also led to understand it was a computer problem. Had it been daytime, with senior staff at hand both at the company and at ATC, the pilots might have been better advised.

On a sophisticated aircraft with so much run by computer, it is too easy to attribute a real problem to the computer, as happened when Captain Piché started transferring fuel to the side from which it was leaking and had to glide eighty miles to salvation.

Some accounts say the pilots were sensibly using their radio altimeter to go back to Lima, but the following cockpit voice recorder (CVR) transcript does not seem to bear this out.

29:49 Captain:

How can it be flying at this speed if we are going down with all the power cut off?

29:56 First officer to ATC:

Can you tell me the altitude please?
Because we have the climb that doesn't...?

29:59 Captain:

Nine.

30:00 GPWS:

Too low! Terrain! Too low, terrain! Too low, terrain!
[These warnings continue until aircraft inverts at 30:50 with the radio altimeter facing the sky.]

30:01 ATC Lima:

Yes, you keep nine seven hundred (9,700) according to presentation, sir.

30:04 First officer to ATC:

Nine seven hundred?

30:09 ATC Lima:

Yes, correct. What is the indicated altitude on board? Have you any visual reference?

30:12 To ATC:

Nine seven hundred, but it indicates "Too low, terrain!"
... Are you sure you have us on the radar at fifty miles?

30:21 Captain:

Hey, look ... With 370 we have ... have ...
[Presumably, the captain was referring to the airspeed indicated by his instruments.]

30:29 First officer:

Have what? 370 of what?

30:36 First officer:

Do we lower the gear?

30:38 Captain:
> *But what do we do with the gear?*
> *Don't know . . . that.*

30:40 [Sound of impact.]
30:41 First officer to ATC:
> *We are hitting water.*

30:44 First officer:
> *Pull it up.*

30:48 Captain:
> *I have it, I have it!*

30:50 GPWS:
> *. . . Too low, terrain! . . .*

[The ground proximity warning system (GPWS) voice alert ceases, because the bottom of the aircraft is no longer facing the sea below but sideways.]
30:55 Captain:
> *We are going to invert!* [Go upside down.]

30:57
> *Whoop! Whoop! Pu—* [Voice alert sounds.]

30:59 Sound of impact.

End of recording, with barometric altimeters indicating 9,700 feet.

All on board—sixty-one passengers and nine crew—lost their lives.

The FDR showed the 757 was traveling at 260 knots and descending at an angle of ten degrees when the left wingtip and left engine pod first snagged the water. Ingestion of water no doubt led to failure of that engine.

With the right engine already at a low power setting because the pilots thought they were flying too fast, their airspeed would have fallen quickly to stalling speed as the aircraft "bounced" and rose to two hundred feet, before inverting and falling back into the sea.

A lawyer made much ado of the suffering the passengers endured in the half hour preceding the impact with the sea. Though the constant changes in speed and height as the pilots responded to the continuous false alerts must have been scary, they can hardly have been expecting to fly straight into the sea.

A judge ordered Aeroperú and the two-dollar-per-hour aircraft polisher who had left the masking tape on the pitot probes and static inlets to pay $29 million to the families of the seventy dead. Another judge had already sentenced the hapless worker to two years in jail.

This incident ultimately led to the closure of the airline.

On Taking Over Control Captain Forgot Timer (Busan, 2002)
Never done circular approach there, even in simulator

Air China, the flag carrier of the People's Republic of China, had an impeccable safety record—forty-seven years without a fatal accident. This was partly because it was able to refuse to fly in adverse weather conditions.

Air China Flight 129, April 15, 2002

The Boeing 767 on the flight from Beijing to Busan, in South Korea, was seventeen years old and not equipped with the enhanced ground proximity warning system (EGPWS), which, besides warning pilots when getting too near the ground immediately below tells them if they are in danger of hitting rising ground *ahead* of them.

Weather at Busan was cloudy and misty, and as the 767 came in to land the controller advised them that a change of wind direction meant that instead of coming straight in, as they first planned, they would have to make a circular approach and land on the runway from the opposite direction.

This was something quite routine and which the pilots should have been prepared for, and that would be included in an approach briefing, in which all eventualities are reviewed, such as having to abort the landing at the last minute because another aircraft is still on the runway.

They came in twenty knots too fast and made a left turn a little late, and not the aggressive, sharp one of forty-five degrees they were supposed to make.

With the extra speed, this meant they were farther along than they should have been and quickly reached the end of the runway, where they were to hold course for precisely twenty seconds before executing a 180-degree base turn to line up with the runway for touchdown.

With the timer set, the copilot remarked that the wind was making the aircraft difficult to handle. At this critical juncture, the captain took over the controls without allotting tasks, notably specifying who was to keep a watch on the timer.

There was some confusion, with the captain flying straight on, although the timer was already showing twenty-five seconds—five seconds beyond the point they should have made their turn.

Flying into cloud, they had lost sight of the runway and should anyway have executed a go-around, since a circular approach is visual, and the runway must therefore always be in sight. Well past the point he would have been after the time was up, the captain began the 180-degree turn, allowing the aircraft to sink below the minimum safe height, which the copilot duly brought to his attention.

Copilot:

Pull up! Pull up!

But it was too late. The aircraft plowed into trees near the top of a mountain. The tail hit first, as the aircraft was pitching up as the pilots tried to save it—though in landing configuration with little thrust, there was little hope of that.

Perhaps because the tall trees cushioned the impact, 37 of the 166 people on board survived, including the captain.

He was interviewed many times but never explained why he had not done a go-around on being unable to see the runway.

Apart from that gross error, a whole series of factors contributed to the crash. The pilots had never done a circular approach to that airport either for real in better visibility or in the simulator.

Of course, local knowledge would have helped, since they would have been aware that one should never go beyond the expressway, as quite high mountains lay behind it.

Air China now class Busan's Gimhae Airport as one needing special care. As airliners always approached from the south, the charts did not show the area to the north with the mountains.

Having only practiced circular approaches at Peking Airport, which is surrounded by low terrain, the pilots may not have been sufficiently aware of the potential dangers, such as at Busan with its mountains. Another factor was work overload due to unpreparedness.

Though captains often do take over in a crisis, this can be dangerous if there is no time before a life or death action is required.

Had BA's Captain Burkill taken over in those final few seconds when his Boeing 777 lost thrust on coming into London's Heathrow airport, the outcome could have been very different. He was (wrongly) criticized by some for that at the time. (See Chapter 2).

Chapter 14
UNIQUE CASES

Without an engineer's understanding of how systems work, pilots have nevertheless at times been tempted to experiment or try out their own "clever" ways to solve a problem. While obvious with hindsight, the outcomes can be unpredictable and sometimes fatal.

Swissair Flight 306, September 4, 1963
Air Florida Flight 90, January 13, 1982
Nigeria Airways Flight 220, July 11, 1991

Taxiing with Brakes on to Clear Fog, Etc. (Zurich, 1963)

Zurich Airport was shrouded in fog at six in the morning when the Swissair Caravelle was due to take off for nearby Geneva before going on to Rome. Despite the poor visibility, controllers let an airport vehicle guide it to the runway.

Finding the fog too thick to take off, the pilots obtained permission to taxi halfway down and back, purportedly to check conditions farther down but in fact to cleverly clear the fog. They would do this by proceeding with the brakes half on and the engines at a higher than usual power to blow the fog away. Having been relatively successful, the pilots duly took off without realizing the Caravelle's brake discs had become extremely hot.

This heat was progressively conducted to the wheel rims, also raising their temperature abnormally. However, it was not until the wheels had been retracted after takeoff that the temperature of the tires and hydraulic lines reached critical levels. At that point the overheated tires exploded, damaging hydraulic lines, causing the fluid to leak and catch fire due to the hot metal. All eighty people on board died in the subsequent crash. They included forty-three children.

Taxiing at high thrust settings with the brakes half on was the cause of the overheating and a tire bursting. However, it was having highly flammable hydraulic fluid that made disaster inevitable.

Air Florida Flight 90 (Washington DC, 1982)

Another example of "clever" unorthodox maneuvers that can be fatal was the Air Florida Flight 90 crash into the icy Potomac River. The captain of the Boeing 737 had "cleverly" used reverse thrust to help the aircraft move back from the stand and then, contrary to instructions for snowy conditions, "cleverly" taxied closely behind another aircraft on the assumption that heat from the engines of that aircraft would help deice his 737.

Using reverse thrust in the presence of snow had sucked it into the engines and following close behind another aircraft would have made the situation worse, since snow on the wings, instead of falling off, would become slush oozing down and freezing on the wings' leading edges and the inlet to the engines. Furthermore, the pilots failed to switch on engine deicing when they came to that point on the checklist, meaning the snow that had been sucked into the engines by reverse thrust froze solid and affected their performance.

Nigeria Airways 2120—Tires on Fire in Wheel Well (July 1991)

Maintenance workers a few days before had decided the Douglas DC-8 jetliner should have its tires replaced, as they were losing pressure. However, the owner, Canadian airline Nationair, which operated it on behalf of Nigeria Airways, stopped them doing that so their flights could run to schedule.

The aircraft made several takeoffs and landings with those low pressures, but when it took off from Jeddah, over the objections of the maintenance engineer, who had been unable to find nitrogen to inflate the tires, to take 257 pilgrims and 14 crew back to Nigeria, the aircraft had to taxi three miles (almost five kilometers) over hot taxiways to the beginning of the runway. The underinflation of the number two tire meant all the weight that axle was meant to support was borne by the number one tire, which flexed beyond normal limits as it rolled, resulting in overheating.

During the takeoff run, the pilots heard the bang as the number one tire failed but continued the run, with the number two tire failing as well. For some reason— perhaps the extreme weight it was bearing—the number two tire ceased rotating. Friction with the runway wore down the rubber and allowed the metal rim to contact the runway.

This metal in turn heated up and no doubt produced sparks, initiating a self-sustaining fire in the wheel well.

Fed by hydraulic fluid and fuel, the blowtorch effect of the slipstream even meant it got hot enough to start burning through the cabin floor. With bodies and seats dropping out, the aircraft crashed short of the runway, killing all on board.

Following this disaster, manufacturers decided to install fire detectors in wheel wells. This incident, caused by cutting corners on maintenance to be more competitive in a difficult market, contributed to the demise of the airline.

Teen Survives Two-Mile Free Fall in Just Her Seat (Peru, 1971)

Dense jungle that broke her fall was almost her undoing

> We describe this event in detail because it is not only remarkable but uplifting, with many valuable lessons regarding the will to survive and human fortitude.
>
> Lansa Flight 508, December 24, 1971

The Lockheed L-188 Electra, the only large turboprop airliner made in the US, had stubby wings and four powerful engines with huge propellers whose prop wash mostly passed over flaps that gave considerable extra wing area when deployed. It was exceptionally good for taking off from short high-altitude runways. In concept it was an excellent aircraft, and it served later as the basic airframe for the Lockheed P3-Orion anti-submarine and maritime surveillance aircraft, of which 650 were produced.

However, a phenomenon called "whirl mode flutter," which was not understood at the time, produced vibrations in the outer engine nacelles that when transmitted to the wings at frequencies coinciding with the harmonics of the outer wing panels would cause the wings to go up and down violently enough to break off.

After a couple of crashes due to loss of a wing, the FAA restricted its speed, until Lockheed eventually solved the problem and modified the wings at great expense. Because of the early crashes, US orders dried up and Lockheed suffered a considerable loss both from cessation of the program and from lawsuits.

It had missed the window of opportunity, since faster, pure-jet aircraft, such as the 727 and 737, were in the offing.

Existing aircraft were in many cases sold abroad, including to South America, where they performed admirably on some routes for years. The rigid wings were not particularly resistant to exceptional stresses, though many were subsequently reinforced.

Christmas Eve Flight

It is alleged the LANSA Lockheed L-188A Electra that took off at midday on Christmas Eve, 1971, from Lima, on Peru's coast, was an early production model and an amalgam of several aircraft. It was to make the short flight inland over the Andes and then the Peruvian rain forest to its first stop, Pucallpa, before going on to Iquitos, even farther inland.

There were ninety-two people on board—eighty-six passengers and six crew. Flying at an altitude of twenty-one thousand feet in good weather, the pilots were musing about how concerned they were about getting back to Lima in time to celebrate Christmas with their families, especially as the flight was already seven hours late.

For twenty-five minutes everything was fine, but then it became increasingly cloudy, and a storm front could be seen ahead even by the passengers. No doubt because they were determined to avoid further delay, the pilots flew straight into it. The clouds became almost black, and passed by the windows, as the passenger who survived said, "like menacing living creatures."

There was extreme turbulence, accompanied by lightning. It got worse, with Christmas presents falling from the overhead bins. Finally, a lightning bolt struck the right engine, and fuel in the wing caught fire. The aircraft dived vertically, with the pilots struggling for control, at which point the rigid wing broke off.

With passengers screaming, the fuselage fell almost vertically, with objects inside tumbling forward, and then broke.

The Search

Aircraft were unable to locate the wreckage, which was obscured by the canopy of tall trees. Also, the torrential rain meant there were no plumes of smoke.

The authorities were inundated with erroneous reports of locations of the crash, perhaps in part because the storm had created sounds and flashes suggestive of a crash. There were so many that the police commander said anyone reporting further sites would be arrested, which obviously put a damper on the flow of information. One of the reports had been correct but was ignored.

Miraculous Free Fall

There were some survivors, but they died before rescuers reached them more than ten days later, guided to the spot, unbelievably, by a passenger thrown from the aircraft who had miraculously survived the two-mile (three-kilometer) free fall.

That person was seventeen-year-old Juliane Koepcke, a half-Peruvian, half-German high school senior studying in Lima, who had been sitting by a window at the rear with her mother next to her and a heavily built man in the aisle seat.

According to Juliane, when the fuselage broke apart everything went quiet, and she found herself alone, with only the sound of wind in her ears. Her mother and the man in the aisle seat gone, she was falling to earth alone, strapped in at the end of her row of seats.

Losing and regaining consciousness, she saw the forest below moving in circles like "green cauliflower, like broccoli" as she fell toward it, pinned painfully in place by her seat belt biting into her stomach.

She only really came to at nine o'clock the following morning, meaning she had remained comatose and in shock the whole afternoon and night. There was no sign of anyone else. No debris.

She had a broken collar bone, a gash in her calf, a deep puncture wound, abrasions of varying severity, concussion, and an eye injury brought about by the change in air pressure.

Having lost her glasses, she found it difficult to see distant objects anyway. She had also lost a shoe and would have to put the foot with the remaining shoe forward every time there was something in the water potentially dangerous.

She was wearing a short skirt that did little to protect her from the cold at night and from mosquito and insect bites, and which a Peruvian newspaper later drew alluringly in a comic strip depicting her ordeal.

She was totally alone, injured, in a dense jungle, and danger lurked everywhere. However, Juliane had several things in her favor:

1. Her parents had inculcated the notion that solutions could always be found, provided one thought calmly and logically;

2. From an early age, she had spent several periods at her father's research station in the rain forest, even going on trips with her parents deep into it with no handholding. She had learnt about piranhas (only dangerous in still water), stingrays, snakes, caimans, poisonous stonefish, and other dangers, including certain plants.

3. Most importantly, her father had taught her that if lost she should look for a stream and follow that, as it would lead her to a river and eventually people.

She shouted to no avail and wandered around in the hope of finding her mother, until finally finding a stream and following it to a creek. She only had boiled sweets to eat, which soon ran out.

Thinking back later, she believed the muddy matter she took in when drinking from the stream and river must have provided some sustenance, as well as hepatitis. On the fourth day, she heard the flapping of large wings that could be only those of vultures.

She thought they might be preying on the dead from the aircraft, which was not far from the truth, as around the next bend she saw a row of seats. The three occupants, two men and a woman, were upside down with their feet sticking up grotesquely in the air, their heads buried deep in the ground. She looked around but could not find any sign of people.

On the fifth or sixth day, she heard the call of hoatzin (stink birds), and, having been told by her ornithologist mother that they are usually associated with open expanses of water, she felt more confident. However, just ahead, where the creek should feed into the river, the way was blocked by impenetrable vegetation.

With tremendous effort she forced her way through the thickets to the side in the direction of the sound of the birds and finally reached the river. Weak and hungry, she half swam, half floated down the moving water in the middle, encountering caimans and dodging logs that could have broken her bones.

As evening approached on the tenth day, she flopped down on a gravel bank and dozed off. When she opened her eyes, she thought she must be dreaming, for a boat was moored nearby.

She swam over to it. It was real; moreover, a path with foot marks led from it to a primitive shelter, which in her weakened state took her hours to crawl to. In it was the outboard motor for the boat and a can of gasoline, some of which she poured onto her maggot-infested wounds, another trick her father had taught her.

She later told London's *Daily Mail* that thirty-five worms came out of her arms alone.

Only the next day at dusk did three forest workers return to the shelter by pure chance as the weather looked bad. Fortunately, she was able to explain in Spanish who she was, as, shocked by her completely bloodshot eyes, they thought she was the water goddess. They tended her as best they could, giving her food, she could hardly get down. Two more men arrived out of the darkness, and after a night with all of them together on the hard shelter floor—she did not dare say she was more comfortable on the ground outside—they took her back to civilization in the boat.

She was able to explain where the crash site was, as the creek she had followed, Stingray Creek, was the only one blocked at the junction with the river by vegetation. When rescue crews following her clues finally located the aircraft, they discovered that as many as fourteen others had initially survived the crash but, unable to seek help, had died awaiting rescue.

Juliane Attributed Her Surviving the Fall to a Combination of:

1. A powerful updraft produced by the storm;
2. Her sitting very tightly buckled in at the end of the seat bench, which meant it was spinning around the heavier end like a maple leaf. Though not conscious for the entire fall, she remembered the jungle below seeming to come toward her, moving in circles;
3. The seat was underneath her, with her facing upwards, so when it hit, it went through the foliage, protecting her like a boat in water;
4. Luckily coming down between high trees linked by lianas, which are long, woody vines that use trees to climb up to the forest canopy to access sunlight.

In her book, she said that a man working on the recovery of the bodies told her the only well-preserved seat bench he found was in a spot between giant trees connected by a dense network of lianas.

The investigation concluded the crash was due to pilot error. They had flown into the storm, and their maneuvers following the lightning strike, which must have weakened the wing, very likely overstressed it.

Rogue Controller Deletes Data (JFK, 1979 or 1980)

As Soviet airliner lands with Soviet ambassador

> One should not forget that air traffic controllers, like bank
> staff, are vulnerable or might have their own agendas.

A report we found on the Internet, dated Thursday, January 31, 1980, that we have been unable to retrieve again to attribute properly and headlined "FAA Acts to Remove a Controller" said:

The Federal Aviation Administration moved yesterday to dismiss an air traffic controller for allegedly tampering with radar data and contributing to the "potential endangerment" of a Soviet airliner being guided to a landing at Kennedy International Airport last January.

The announcement of the FAA action said that "important flight data" on the Soviet plane, a four-jet Ilyushin 62 operated by the airline Aeroflot, had been "deliberately erased" as the aircraft approached Kennedy. Among those on board the plane was the Soviet ambassador to the United States, Anatoly F. Dobrynin.

There are ways a rogue controller—or worse, controllers acting in unison—could put aircraft in great danger, but no more will be said, as the author does not want this to become a terrorist's handbook.

Radar Facilities Vulnerable

However, facilities linked to air traffic control probably need protecting and backups.

For example, many years ago in Japan, some activists managed to find out where the cables linking ground radar facilities passed underground and brought down Tokyo's ATC system by cutting them.

The American Airlines Flight 965 disaster at Cali would more than likely not have happened had the radar installation not been blown up by FARC antigovernment fighters, and the air traffic controller had been able to see the aircraft.

747's Terrifying Thirty-Thousand-Foot Plunge (Pacific, 1985)
Mistakes led to upset, then pilot saved them twice over

> An airliner is somewhat like a two-legged human walking assuredly and stably. All is fine until either trip up—the fall can be precipitous and recovery not easy. However, airliners often have much more height to play with.
>
> China Airlines Flight 006, February 19, 1985

China Airlines, with the call sign "Dynasty," is not the flagship airline of the People's Republic of China but that of the offshore island Taiwan.

Their flight from Taiwan to Los Angeles was the regularly scheduled one in a Boeing 747SP (special performance), designed for what at the time were considered ultra-long-haul flights. For such a long flight there were two crews, but the captain and first officer from the primary crew were back in their seats as it approached the US coast, with the captain having returned early from his rest, saying he had found it difficult to sleep.

Coffin Corner

Everything was going smoothly, with the performance management system and autopilot maintaining the aircraft on its course at Mach 0.85. They were flying in what is referred to as "coffin corner," namely at a considerable height, where there is relatively little margin between going too fast and too slow.

Going too fast would mean air passing some parts of the aircraft would exceed the speed of sound (Mach 1) thus producing shock waves. Going too slowly in the thin air would cause the aircraft to stall.

Normally, with the autothrust constantly making minor adjustments, this posed no problem, though the pilots would always be aware that maintaining the correct airspeed was essential.

As they approached reporting point Redo, about 300 nautical miles (550 kilometers) northwest of San Francisco, they encountered some clear air turbulence, which very fortunately, as proved later, prompted the captain to tell the passengers to fasten their seat belts. As the airspeed fluctuated between Mach 0.84 (251 KIAS) and Mach 0.88 (264 KIAS), the autothrottle moved the throttles forward and aft to maintain the commanded cruise Mach number of 0.85.

When the airspeed again rose to Mach 0.88, the autothrottle reduced power, and then when the airspeed fell to Mach 0.84 immediately applied more. Engines one, two, and three responded, while engine number four did not. The flight engineer moved the throttle for that engine back and forth, with no perceptible response, until it flamed out.

The captain asked for the performance charts to ascertain the three-engine en route cruise altitude and told the first officer to request permission from air traffic control for them to fly at a lower altitude. The flight engineer began going through the checklist in preparation for a restart at lower altitude but was cut short by the captain ordering him to restart it immediately, even though doing so was virtually impossible at that altitude and contrary to SOP (standard operating procedure), which said a restart should only be attempted below thirty thousand feet.

The Boeing 747 can fly perfectly well on three engines and easily stay up with two, so this was by no means a crisis and indeed something that happened from time to time. However, with one engine, and particularly an outboard one, not working, thrust was asymmetric, with the aircraft so much wanting to yaw to the right that application of the rudder was required to compensate.

The autopilot on the 747, unlike the Airbus A330, had no control over the rudder, as moving the ailerons was largely sufficient for making normal turns and compensating for any yaw. The autopilot was therefore struggling to keep the aircraft on course, and even with the control column controlling the ailerons hard over to the left, the aircraft was tipping and turning to the right.

Instead of immediately taking over manual control, the captain concerned himself with the restarting the number four engine—something as said was impossible at that great height. With one less engine, the aircraft was losing speed and descending into the clouds.

When the captain belatedly assumed manual control, the right bank had already reached a precarious sixty degrees, and since he failed to apply left rudder and was ill prepared, the aircraft lurched even farther to the right and tipped downward. So focused was he on his airspeed that he did not monitor the attitude indicator, and when he turned his attention to it, he found it unbelievable— something he had never seen, as in a 747 the maximum might be forty-five degrees, and they were way beyond that—and exclaimed it had failed. Faced with all the attitude indicators showing what they thought were "crazy" readings, the crew believed they had failed, something highly improbable.

The Upset

In cloud and without recourse to their attitude indicators, the pilots were at a loss as the aircraft plunged downward.

The terrifying drop was in two parts, with the second part worse than the first. The first part, a 10,310-foot descent to 30,132 feet in thirty-three seconds, where the aircraft seemed to stabilize somewhat, and the second part, from 30,132 feet to 9,577 feet in one minute fifty-two seconds of greater hell.

The 747 had broken out of the clouds at 11,000 feet (3,400 meters), allowing the captain to see the horizon and, by surprising airmanship, bring the plane under control, leveling out at 9,600 feet (2,900 meters). However, this subjected the passengers to tremendous g-forces. Engines one, two, and three, which the crew had mistakenly assumed had flamed out, appeared to be working again, the problematic engine number four restarted.

With all four engines working normally, and the aircraft seeming to be in good order, they sought permission to climb and proceed to Los Angeles. However, the inboard main landing gear was down and could not be retracted because of failure in one of the hydraulic systems.

The extra drag meant they would not have enough fuel (and reserves) to reach Los Angeles, so they requested permission to land at San Francisco and were allotted a straight-in landing, which was fortunate, as the elevators in the tail had been compromised, probably by part of the main wheel bay, which was blown off when the aircraft exceeded its maximum airspeed during the drop.

By another dint of good airmanship, the captain brought the 747 in to a perfect touchdown, adjusting engine power to control the rate and angle of descent.

All 251 passengers and 23 crew had survived, with 22 minor injuries and two serious casualties, one of whom was a male flight attendant, who spent just over two days in hospital with acute back strain, while the other was a passenger with lacerations and bone fractures on his right foot.

Serious injuries are officially defined as:

Any injury which

(1) requires hospitalization for more than forty-eight hours, commencing within seven days from the date the injury was received;

(2) results in a fracture of any bone (except simple fractures of fingers, toes, or nose).

Passengers Terrified

This must have been one of the most frightening passenger experiences ever.

With the aircraft diving vertically and at various angles, and unattached passengers and flight attendants floating to the ceiling at times or pressed down or up with forces reaching 5 g at others.

It was so traumatic that some could not remember the details when interviewed; others cite the odor of urine and food, as noodles and dishes flew around, since smells link one to events.

While mentally passengers were certain they were going to die, physically they were like astronauts under training being given the experience of weightlessness with no hard impacts. Compared with passengers hitting the ceiling panels on other airliners caught up in clear turbulence, it was relatively benign, though the fact that so many had their seat belts fastened helped considerably.

Damage to the Aircraft

Damage to the aircraft caused by the overspeed and parts breaking off and striking others was much greater than the pilots realized.

For instance, the elevators in the tail had been struck by the broken-off cover of the main wheel bay. With a large segment missing, the captain had had to land the aircraft by varying engine power to adjust the pitch on coming in to land.

The wings were bent permanently two to three inches upward at the wingtips, but within the manufacturer's allowable tolerances. This may seem a lot, but in view of the length of the wings did not represent a great degree of distortion. Indeed, after repairs, the aircraft remained in service with the company for more than eleven years before being transferred to other owners.

The Investigation

To protect pilot privacy, the cockpit voice recording was overwritten every thirty minutes, so there was nothing of relevance left when power was switched off on arrival in San Francisco. Investigators had to fall back on interviews with the aircrew. While the cockpit data recorder proved most helpful, unraveling it took considerable time, as there were gaps where it had undergone the exceptional g-forces during the precipitous descent.

The near calamity had been so unnecessary, for if the captain had followed standard operating procedure and descended to thirty thousand feet before trying to restart the number four engine, there would have been no problem.

He had never experienced an in-flight engine failure, though had coped with one on takeoff in the simulator. Although not mentioned in the official report, it is alleged elsewhere that he was not aware that the autopilot had no effect on the rudder.

However, the Boeing training manual for the 747 had very precise instructions regarding the actions to be taken in the event of an engine failure, with particular regard to the use of the rudder and the setting of the rudder trim so the aircraft would fly straight without recourse to use of the ailerons. Since the captain had so many flying hours (15,494, of which 3,748 were in Boeing 747s), those training manual instructions were possibly a distant memory.

The investigators concluded rather that the captain's initial mistakes were due to fatigue (which he himself would not admit) as it was his natural time for sleeping and in the days prior to the flight he had flown several sectors in different time zones.

Though the precipitating factor was the hanging of the number four engine, the probable cause of this incident was the captain's preoccupation with an inflight malfunction and his failure to monitor properly the airplane's flight instruments, which resulted in his losing control of the airplane. The contributing factor was the captain relying for too long on the autopilot instead of getting the feel of the aircraft early on before things got out of hand.

747 Cargo Hold Door Opens Midflight (Honolulu, 1989)

Nine business class passengers ejected

> Highlighted the danger of investigators concluding "the most probable cause" is the cause.
>
> United Airlines Flight 811, February 24, 1989

The aircraft used for United Airlines Flight UA811, from Honolulu to Auckland, New Zealand, on February 24, 1989, with 337 passengers on board, was an old Boeing 747 that had seen considerable service.

Honolulu was essentially a refueling stop—the airline also had a nonstop flight from Los Angeles to Auckland, for which they used a newer long-range 747.

The aircraft received clearance to take off at 1:52 a.m. local time and climbed out as usual, except for deviating somewhat from the normal course to avoid some thunderstorm cells, their presence ultimately proving fortunate, as they made the captain keep the "Fasten Seat Belt!" signs switched on.

Sixteen minutes into the flight, with the aircraft having passed twenty-two thousand feet on its climb to its thirty-thousand-plus cruising height for the long transpacific leg to Auckland, the aircraft juddered, and the aircrew heard a thud that appeared to have come from behind and below them. There followed a tremendous explosion, which for a moment tilted the aircraft leftward.

Situation in The Aircraft

The roar of the wind became unbelievably loud, and the misting of the air confirmed that the aircraft had suffered a rapid decompression. Failure of the lights added to the fears of many that this was to be another Lockerbie.

However, the emergency lighting soon kicked in, and people began to realize the aircraft was not—at least for the time being—in the process of breaking up. The cabin pressure warning horn prompted the crew to put on their oxygen masks, but to their consternation they found there appeared to be no oxygen.

In putting the aircraft into an emergency dive to get to a level where they could breathe more easily, the captain might, as in the Aloha case, have been putting the integrity of the aircraft at risk. At the time, there was no way he could have known the extent of the damage. In fact, even without an emergency dive the flight crew should have been able to stay operational until reaching a reasonably comfortable height.

The first officer entered 7700 (the emergency code) into the transponder and called Honolulu Approach Control to formalize the emergency.

While able to communicate with far-off ATC, the pilots could not communicate with the cabin crew just behind them. Meanwhile, the instruments were showing the number three engine was failing and would have to be shut down. After that was completed, the flight engineer went back to inspect the damage.

In the early 747s, the upper cabin behind the flight deck was quite small. The engineer was astounded to see a three-meter-wide section of the skin below the windows had separated from the stringers and formers on the right-hand side and open sky visible between the gaps. This accounted for the noise of the wind in the cockpit.

Worse was to come.

On descending to the larger lower-deck business-class cabin below, the flight engineer saw that there the stringers and formers had disappeared as well, leaving a three-meter-wide gaping hole extending from floor level to the ceiling. What was more, the floor had failed just above the cargo hold door below, and the five rows of twin seats that had been attached to it there had disappeared, presumably together with a number of passengers, as the aircraft had been quite full.

The remaining business-class passengers had tried to move back to the main cabin, where the scene was almost unimaginable. People were screaming, some were hysterical, and others were already in the brace position, waiting for the aircraft to crash. Because the volume of air in the main passenger cabins had been so much greater, the effect of the mass of air rushing forward when the sudden decompression occurred had been even greater too. The escaping air had hurled meal trays and glasses with such force that some were even embedded in the bulkheads. It had also dislodged wall and ceiling panels, and there was dust and debris everywhere.

The projectiles had injured a number of passengers, and even those who were unscathed seemed distressed because of the wind and the stress.

The cabin crew valiantly tried to get the situation in hand, but the noise of the wind made communication with the passengers virtually impossible. One positive was that having descended to a lower altitude, the passengers, whose oxygen masks were not working, were coping.

In assessing the damage, the flight engineer was particularly concerned to see long streaks of flame emanating sporadically from the number four engine (the one on the extreme right). The violence of the decompression had ejected debris, or possibly a passenger, not only into the number three engine, which had been shut down, but even as far as the outboard engine. Hurrying back to the flight deck, the flight engineer found his colleagues waiting for him to assist with the shutdown of that engine, which they duly carried out.

With engine power on only one side, the 747 limped back toward Honolulu, with the reduced speed having somewhat lessened the disturbing noise of the wind. Twenty minutes later the distraught and terrified passengers had their spirits raised by the sight of Honolulu, which they had left shortly before.

When the pilots lowered the flaps to land, a flap asymmetry appeared, and the captain had to limit the amount of flap to ten degrees.

He decided to come in at 190 to 200 knots not only because of the limited amount of flap, but also because the aircraft might be difficult to control at the normal lower speed due to damage to some control surfaces, having both engines on one side shut down, and the gaping hole.

He made a perfect landing and managed to bring the aircraft safely to a halt using the wheel brakes and idle reverse thrust on the two good engines.

The captain ordered an emergency evacuation, in the course of which some passengers—and surprisingly, it is said, all the cabin crew—sustained some form of injury.

A number of the passengers had been injured when the decompression occurred.

Nine business-class passengers had been ejected altogether—eight in the seats they were sitting in and the ninth, who had been sitting just across the aisle from that block of seats, without his seat, making one wonder whether he was properly strapped in.

Things could have been much worse, and the fact that the aircraft remained intact is perhaps a credit to Boeing, especially as it was an early-model 747. Both the flight crew and the cabin crew performed well in very difficult circumstances. Valuable lessons were learned, such as ensuring the pilots and cabin crew are guaranteed to have oxygen available; the oxygen requirement is much greater for someone engaged in mental activity as well as physical.

The Investigation

It was immediately obvious that the untoward opening of the cargo hold door on the front right-hand side was responsible for the explosive decompression and associated structural damage. Cargo hold doors, as in the case of those on the DC-10, have often been problematic on high-flying jets as in order to leave more room for cargo they often open outwards, unlike the plug doors in the passenger cabins that seal more tightly the higher the aircraft.

An extremely complicated mechanism, consisting of pushrods, cranks, cams, and latches to mention only a few of the items, is required to cope with the width. In addition, on large aircraft an electric motor is usually incorporated to do the basic locking and unlocking, with manual locks completing the process. There should be no danger of the unlocking function operating in flight, as the motor uses electrical power only available on the ground either from the APU (auxiliary power unit) at the rear of the aircraft, or from the airport electricity supply.

NTSB's Wrong Conclusion

Without the actual door, the NTSB felt they had to surmise what happened and produced a report concluding that since, in their view, a normal door could not open in flight, the locking mechanism must have been damaged by poor ground handling as alleged occurred in the case of a cargo hold door on a 747 that took off from London's Heathrow in 1987.

Parents of Victim Pursue Their Own Investigation

It is rare for relatives of victims to have any voice in accident investigations, let alone carry out their own investigation. Yet this is what happened here, leading to the NTSB revising its conclusions.

Kevin and Susan Campbell, parents of Lee Campbell who was one of the passengers sucked out of the business class cabin—they expressed the hope he was sucked into the inboard engine and did not have to suffer the long fall to earth—followed the investigation from the outset.

Having money and time, they not only went to Honolulu and but travelled the country to get technical information and badgered the NTSB. When the latter held a public meeting to explain their conclusion that the door had been damaged by poor ground handling the Campbell's were incensed. When told they could take some documentation, they in doing so scooped up a considerable amount of material intended for the NTSB's internal use. This provided many useful leads, enabling them to finally persuade the NTSB Board to reconsider and prove the matter one way or the other by retrieving the door.

The incident had occurred in February 1989, and in September the following year by an incredible feat of technology the US Navy recovered the cargo door (in two pieces) from a depth of 14,200 feet. The recovered door showed it had been unlocked electrically and the manual locking pins had insufficient strength to prevent the door opening.

This contradicted the April 1990 NTSB report, which concluded the electrical unlocking of the door prior to takeoff could only be considered a remote possibility.

This shows the danger, in the absence of definitive evidence, of assuming without any proof that what was the most probable cause by far was the cause.

The NTSB published a correction.

Improvements, too late for those nine business-class passengers, were subsequently made, and there has not been an accident since due to the opening of a Boeing 747 cargo door.

China Airlines and El Al 747F Engine Mounts (1991 and 1992)

Boeing redesigns engine mounts at great expense

> It is not so widely known that Boeing spent a considerable amount of money redesigning the engine-supporting pylons on its early 747s and refitting many aircraft following two crashes of the cargo versions.
>
> China Airlines 747 Freighter, December 29, 1991
> El Al 747 Freighter, October 4, 1992

The supporting pylons for engines mounted under the wings of airliners are usually designed to allow the engine to possibly fall off in certain circumstances, such as when exceptional torque is produced by an engine seizing up; when an engine is seriously on fire; and when ditching in water, so the wing is not torn off, or so the aircraft does not spin around disastrously and cartwheel.

China Airlines Freighter 747

On December 29, 1991, the inboard number three engine came off an eleven-year-old China Airlines Boeing 747-2R7F freighter as it was climbing out under high power from Taiwan's Chiang Kai-Shek International Airport. Because it was under high power the engine initially shot forward before falling back and glancing off the outboard number four engine set farther back, which in turn also fell off. The aircraft subsequently crashed, killing all five occupants.

Though the number three engine was retrieved from the sea some distance from the main debris, the pylon was only discovered seven months later.

El Al Freighter 747

Nine months after that disaster, exactly the same thing happened to an El Al Cargo 747 climbing out of Amsterdam's Schiphol Airport. Besides knocking off the outboard engine the number three engine took away a large section of the leading edge of the wing. The captain just about managed to keep the aircraft under control with limited aileron function and were able to fly on. However, when they slowed the aircraft to return to the airport to make an emergency landing, the damaged wing stalled, and the aircraft rolled over very much like the DC-10 did on slowing after losing an engine at Chicago. The aircraft plowed into an eleven-story apartment complex in Amsterdam's down-market district of Bijlmer.

The last words from the crew were disturbingly matter of fact:

Going down . . . eh . . . 1862, going down, going down. Copied, going down?

In addition to the four occupants of the aircraft, forty-seven people were killed on the ground, with the total perhaps more, as the building housed a number of unregistered illegal immigrants. The disaster immediately received considerable publicity, because the dramatic pictures probably made people consider just how much damage an aircraft plunging into a building can cause.

The mystery surrounding the nature of the aircraft's cargo was to give the story legs.

Amsterdam's Schiphol Airport was one of several European airports allowing El Al to transship cargo unsupervised, and as a result the details of the manifest were not public knowledge. After claiming the freighter had been carrying innocuous flowers and perfume, the Israeli government eventually admitted that a precursor for making nerve gas (sarin) had been on board, but claimed it was for testing filters, and the amount was small.

It was a very sensitive matter, especially as the aircraft had come from the United States and it would look bad if the Americans were seen to be providing Israel with materials for chemical warfare. Depleted uranium was also present but could have been from the aircraft itself to add stabilizing weight to certain parts.

Residents reported seeing men in white suits sifting through the wreckage.

People, and notably rescuers in the area of the crash, where the debris burned for an hour and smoldered for several more, reported all sorts of ailments and depression, and there were accusations of a cover-up. As in the case of 9/11, people would anyway have been affected by the untold number of constituents in the cloud of smoke and dust when an aircraft, laden with fuel just after takeoff, hits a building.

The nature of the cargo is not very relevant here, except to remark that some very nasty things probably pass over our heads, sometimes in diplomatic bags.

A fourteen-inch crack was found in one of the fuse pins used for attaching the engines on the El Al freighter and designed to shear as a safety measure under the special circumstances mentioned above, but not in normal service. Such cracks can develop when metal is under repetitive flexing conditions, especially if there is an initial pit on the surface due to corrosion, in a phenomenon called *stress-assisted corrosion*, where the stress facilitates the penetration of the corrosion. The initial pit would probably have been due to the surface being left vulnerable to corrosion (passive) due to lack of primer or faulty coating during manufacture. Incidentally, shortly before, Boeing had issued warnings concerning the pins used for attaching the Pratt & Whitney engines in question.

Following these two incidents, Boeing notified users about the necessary checks and then redesigned the entire mounting system. Modifying existing aircraft cost the company a considerable amount of money, as it involved a lengthy task, said by one commentator to be forty days. In addition, a considerable number of susceptible 747s had been delivered.

This accident with so few people on board made the Boeing 747 safer; unfortunately, there were ten times more victims on the ground.

Siting or expanding airports where aircraft have to overfly cities is obviously not ideal.

In-Flight Deployment of Thrust Reversers (Lauda Air and TAM)
Only meant for slowing aircraft on the ground

> In-flight deployment of a thrust reverser, especially when the engines are at high-power settings, can be disastrous. You have one engine pushing the aircraft forward and the one on the other wing pulling it backward.
>
> Lauda Air 004, May 26, 1991
> TAM Flight 402, October 31, 1996

Lauda Air 004

Start-up airlines on long-distance routes with, say, less than half a dozen sizable aircraft are loath to take any out of service for nonessential checking, as, with no replacement, this can mean canceling flights or even services outright. For instance, when a Lauda Air 767 crashed in Thailand on its way back to Vienna, the airline lost a quarter of its capacity and had to temporarily cancel some services to Australia.

Though not mentioned in the TV documentary *Mayday*, featuring and indeed eulogizing the airline's founder, Niki Lauda, sixty-one error messages concerning that 767's thrust reverser were found in its computer. Even though there was a Boeing representative at Lauda Air's Vienna home base, he was not consulted.

The 767, with 213 passengers and 10 crew, had taken off for Vienna from Bangkok's Don Mueang Airport at 23:02 local time. Four minutes later the pilots received a visual warning concerning the thrust reverser on the left-hand engine, but their documentation said it was just advisory, perhaps meaning there could be problems with it on landing, and they continued regardless. Eleven minutes later, with the copilot saying the reverser had deployed, the aircraft tipped to the left and plunged downward so fast that it broke up at about four thousand feet and came down in an isolated mountainous area six hundred meters above sea level. Debris was spread over a square kilometer of forest. There could be no survivors.

The Thais sent in their own investigators, and they were joined by a team from the NTSB led by Bob MacIntosh, who found that local people were removing items that could be essential for the inquiry. The black boxes were found, but the cockpit data recorder was too damaged by fire to be of any use; however, the voice recorder could be read.

The left engine was found with the thrust reverser obviously deployed, so with confirmation from the voice recorder that it had been, there was no doubt that was the cause of the crash. But without the data recorder evidence, and with the wiring either burned or stolen, there was no way to determine why it had deployed.

To obtain certification from the FAA, Boeing had tried deploying the thrust reverser in flight and found recovery possible, but it was later found this had been with a pilot expecting it and at the relatively low airspeed of 250 knots.

Acknowledging such an occurrence could be fatal at higher speed or when unexpected, Boeing sent telexes to all users and incorporated extra safety devices, such as locks, not only on the 767 but also on other aircraft.

TAM Flight 402

The Brazilian TAM air crash occurred five years later, when manufacturers were much more aware of the danger of in-flight deployment of a thrust reverser. The makers of the popular Fokker 100 twin-jet came up with an ingenious way to ensure that deployment of a thrust reverser, especially on takeoff, would not cripple their aircraft. They simply had a cable link the thrust reverser to the thrust lever so that if it did accidentally deploy it would pull the lever back to cut power to that engine. As twin-jets are designed to be able to easily take off with one engine, there would be no problem.

As the TAM 402 Fokker 100 took off from Sao Paulo, the captain's attention was drawn to a warning that the autothrust was not working properly, in itself not serious enough for him to reject the takeoff, as the levers could be worked manually. Perhaps because of an intermittently faulty micro-switch and a short circuit, the right engine thrust reverser deployed, causing the aircraft to tip and veer to the right, but just when it looked bad the captain regained control thanks to the safety mechanism pulling the throttle back and cutting power to that engine.

However, the copilot, thinking the lever had come back on its own, pushed it forward, and again the aircraft misbehaved before the safety system operated.

The captain, with the autothrottle warnings in his mind, ordered for it to be switched off. The copilot then forcefully held the right-hand throttle lever forward to prevent it returning, putting so much strain on the cable that a link in the middle (placed there so that it could be disconnected for servicing) parted.

The aircraft then plunged, with the right wing down, into a housing area just beyond the airport, killing all ninety-six occupants and, surprisingly, only three people on the ground, despite raging fires from burning fuel.

The aircraft manufacturer had considered such an event so unlikely it did not insist on training for such a mode.

Captain's Son Disengages A310 Autopilot (Russia, 1994)
Pilots fail to notice partial disengagement

> The captain on this flight allowed his teenage son to sit in
> his seat for a moment. Full details only became generally
> available thanks to diligent research by the late Macarthur
> Job and his assistants. The following distillation is based
> (with permission) on his account in *Air Disaster* (Vol. 3).
>
> Aeroflot Flight 593, March 23, 1994

The Aeroflot A310 was on a regular scheduled flight from Moscow to Hong Kong. The three-man flight crew consisted of Captain Danilov, the commander, Captain Kudrinsky, who was the reserve commander, needed for such a long trip, and Second Pilot Piskarev.

In addition, there were sixty-five passengers and nine flight attendants. Among the passengers was an off-duty captain.

The presence in the passenger cabin of Captain Kudrinsky's family, and notably his son, El'dar, fifteen, and daughter, Yana, thirteen, would make the trip more memorable than his usual flights. He would be able to relax with them before being called to the cockpit to take over from Captain Danilov, who was flying the most difficult sectors out of Moscow—near sensitive areas and where there was always considerable traffic.

In accordance with regulations, medical staff at Moscow checked the pilots' blood alcohol levels and blood pressure before the flight, and they recorded "nothing untoward."

The presence of alcohol was not given as a possible contributory factor, though there were suggestions that the captain was drinking with his family. One story said he struggled to get back to the cockpit from the cabin.

When Captain Kudrinsky finally took over from Captain Danilov, with Piskarev still acting as copilot, it seems that the latter, a short man, at some point pushed his seat right back, either to relax after his hard work or to get up for a moment, and left it pushed back.

Just as they were about to pass near the city of Novosibirsk, in the middle of Siberia, Makarov, the off-duty captain, brought the two kids to the cockpit, no doubt knowing it would be the last straightforward sector before crossing the frontier into Mongolia.

Vacating his seat, Captain Kudrinsky allowed his daughter to take his place, adjusting the seat's height so she could see out of the windscreen. He told his daughter to hold the controls and adjusted the heading selector on the autopilot slightly, first in one direction and then in the opposite direction.

In the girl's gentle hands, the control column duly moved as the autopilot banked slightly to adjust the course to the selected heading. The idea was to let her get the feel of flying the aircraft. Evidently not too enthralled, she soon gave up her seat to her eager elder brother.

El'dar took her place, with Makarov filming the event with a video camera. Instead of being passive like his sister, El'dar, having taken in what his father had said about how the controls worked, asked whether he could move the control wheel.

His father said he could, whereupon El'dar sharply turned it three to four degrees to the left before his father could anticipate his move by turning the autopilot heading selector, as he had done for the young girl. Kudrinsky then returned the selector to NAV (automatic navigation) mode, and the aircraft banked the other way to resume its preset track.

Unfortunately, by exerting a very positive force on the control column, the boy had caused the autopilot to disengage in the lateral (banking) axis.

As already mentioned in the context of the TriStar Everglades crash (See previous chapter), manufacturers program autopilots to disengage if a force exceeding a certain limit is applied to the control column so they can take over in an emergency.

This meant that a strong boy with one minute's flying experience and no training, and Piskarev, who was short and had his seat so far back he was almost out of reach of the controls, were the only people controlling the aircraft in the banking (rolling) axis.

At the time the A310 did not have any system, aural or visual, to warn pilots of such an autopilot disconnect, probably because the manufacturer thought it could only happen if a pilot moved the control column sharply, in which case he would know what he had done and would be aware of what was happening. With none of the professional pilots in the cockpit realizing what had happened, El'dar kept pushing the control column (yoke) to the right, perhaps because he was right-handed.

In consequence, the aircraft increased its right-hand bank from fifteen to twenty degrees in seven seconds. However, with Kudrinsky chatting to his daughter, and Piskarev assuming the autopilot was doing everything, no one noticed the gradual increase in bank, which due to the turn it produced would at night only have been evident from the artificial horizon.

With the bank progressively increasing and attaining forty-five degrees forty seconds after Kudrinsky, expecting the aircraft would look after itself, had reset the autopilot to NAV, it was El'dar who realized something odd was happening. He interrupted his father to ask why the aircraft was turning, something he also could only have determined from the instruments.

Asked by his father whether it was turning by itself, El'dar said it was, perhaps not realizing the effect of his hand on the control column.

The three proper pilots then launched into a discussion as to why the autopilot was making the aircraft turn on its own and concluded that it must be a holding pattern. Soon the bank had attained fifty degrees, still without the three pilots realizing anything was amiss.

Pilots, learning to fly on tiny aircraft, know that when an aircraft banks steeply, the amount of lift decreases. In consequence, they increase engine power and raise the nose when doing so to avoid sinking. Likewise, the A310's autopilot increased the engine power and raised the nose in order to maintain its programmed altitude and speed.

It was Makarov, the off-duty captain, no doubt feeling the g-forces on his feet, who noticed something was wrong. No sooner had he uttered a warning than the aircraft, in order to maintain its height, pitched upward. It then began buffeting, a sure sign it was about to stall.

Kudrinsky called out:

Hold the control column. Hold it!

Piskarev immediately turned his control column yoke to the left to counter the increasingly precipitous rightward bank and would no doubt have succeeded in righting the aircraft had El'dar not also followed his father's instructions, probably intended for Piskarev.

Not knowing what action to take, the boy gamely clutched the yoke, maintaining it firmly in an almost neutral position. This resulted in an unequal battle between the boy ensconced in the perfect position and the ill-placed Piskarev. The latter was only five foot three inches (160 centimeters) tall, and with his seat right back, his shoulder harness would be keeping him at arm's length from the control column and unable to reach the rudder pedals.

As a result, Piskarev's efforts were insufficient to halt the dangerously increasing bank, which, by causing the aircraft to lose lift, was making the autopilot raise the nose farther to maintain height. Finally, Piskarev must have knowingly overridden the autopilot by pushing the control column sharply forward, thus causing it to disengage completely.

This time there was an aural warning that the autopilot had disengaged. This was followed first by the nonurgent warning that the aircraft had departed from its designated height and then by the more pressing warning of an imminent stall. With these warnings coming in quick succession and increasing stress levels, all three pilots started shouting conflicting instructions to El'dar.

If the boy had had even minimal flying experience, he might have known instinctively what to do to put the aircraft on a level keel. However, with the general confusion and the situation becoming increasingly scary, there was not much hope. He was probably transfixed.

Meanwhile, the Alpha floor safety function (mentioned in connection with the Habsheim air show Airbus crash) sensed that the aircraft was going into a stall and pushed the nose down by adjusting the tail trim just as Piskarev was trying to do the same by pushing the control column forward. This put the aircraft into a forty-degree dive that was to last thirteen seconds. With the engines still supplying normal cruising thrust, the airspeed continued to build up alarmingly even after the overspeed alarm had sounded.

Piskarev yanked back the control column to pull the aircraft out of its precipitous dive just as Kudrinsky, trying to get back in his seat, was shouting to the boy, "Get out! Get out!" The powerful g-forces resulting from the aircraft beginning to level out multiplied the weight of the boy, making it even more difficult for him to clamber out.

With the aircraft leveling out and going into a climb, Piskarev, no doubt concerned by the overspeed warning, called for the engine thrust to be reduced regardless of the fact that he was holding the control column fully back. Why he kept the control column fully back is difficult to comprehend.

There have even been suggestions that he was using it to pull himself and his seat forward. Meanwhile, the reduction in g-forces had allowed El'dar to vacate his seat and let his father slip in, albeit with it in the back position, which was not to help matters later.

With full-up elevator and airspeed of only ninety-seven knots, the aircraft slewed to the right and then slipped into a downward spin to the left. Belatedly Piskarev asked for full throttle but having the elevators still in the full-up position, this was not destined to help recovery. As the aircraft reached two hundred knots, it went into an uncontrolled spin that was to last for a minute.

With the aircraft in a twenty-degree dive and the fully back control column(s) keeping the aircraft in a semi-stall, Kudrinsky, now back in his seat, was finally managing to get out of the spin using the rudder.

So Near Salvation

They leveled out with only a little over 1,000 feet (350 m) of altitude remaining, which would have been fine had they not at the time been sinking at a rate of 13,870 feet a minute (70 meters a second).

With insufficient time to arrest their descent, they plunged onto the trees on a snow-covered slope of a 2,000-foot (600-meter) hill some three hundred nautical miles southwest of the Siberian capital, Novosibirsk.

Rescuers found the fire and explosion impact had destroyed much of the wreckage—not that anyone could have survived the impact anyway.

Had it not been for a cockpit video recording taken by the off-duty captain, it would not have been possible to determine exactly what happened, and particularly who did what.

Many pilots are against having a video recorder in addition to a voice recorder in the cockpit, even though one would be an invaluable tool for determining what happened in some cases.

Autopilot Takes Unconscious Pilots to Destination (Greece, 2005)

Cabin pressure alarm assumed to be for something else

> Not realizing cabin pressurization was set to "Manual" when they took off, the 737 pilots lost consciousness due to lack of oxygen.
>
> Helios Airways Flight 522, August 14, 2005

At 9:00 a.m. local time, the Helios Airways Boeing 737-300 took off from Larnaca, Cyprus, for Athens, where it was to make a stopover on its way to Prague. On board were 121 people, including the 2 pilots and 4 cabin crew.

As the aircraft climbed through ten thousand feet, the cabin altitude (air pressure) warning horn sounded. As the same warning sound is also used to indicate a configuration mistake, such as failure to extend flaps at takeoff, the pilots assumed it was merely a false alert. They even discussed the problem with their maintenance people at Larnaca, but with some difficulty, as the captain was German, the first officer Cypriot, and the maintenance engineer English.

On the advice of maintenance about how to silence the irritating horn, the captain left his seat to trip the relevant circuit breaker behind his seat, but due to the extra exertion and lack of oxygen, he collapsed before he could do so. The last communication received by ATC was eleven minutes after takeoff as the aircraft was passing through twenty-two thousand feet, the height at which lack of oxygen renders one fully comatose.

The aircraft continued to climb to its cruising height of thirty-four thousand feet and continued toward Athens, as programmed in the flight management control system (FMCS). As it approached their airspace, Greek air traffic controllers were surprised at not being able to communicate but were initially not too concerned, as they had heard about the air-conditioning problem the pilots had mentioned only four minutes after takeoff from Larnaca. Becoming concerned that some sort of hijacking might be involved, they alerted the Greek air force but told them to hold off, thinking the Helios flight was sorting out its technical problems.

Finally, at 10:55 a.m. two air force F-16s were scrambled. On intercepting the aircraft, they reported that the first officer was slumped over his seat and that the captain's seat was unoccupied. They then said two people had entered the cockpit wearing oxygen masks. The pilots also noticed that the passengers' oxygen masks had deployed.

The cockpit voice recorder later showed someone with a very labored male voice had made Mayday calls, which the controllers had not picked up, no doubt because the frequency was still set for the point of departure.

The first thing a professional airline pilot taking over control would have done would have been to bring the aircraft down to a height where breathing would have been easier. However, the pilot in question was flight attendant Prodromou, a private pilot with only a few hours' experience on a Cessna. Being unfamiliar with the 737 controls, he might well have wanted to seek advice over the radio before performing a maneuver from which he might not be able to recover, and there is evidence he hesitated for a long time.

Greek investigators later said Prodromou, together with a female colleague, used an emergency oxygen kit, opened the cockpit door using a code, and managed to fly the plane for ten to twelve minutes before it crashed from lack of fuel.

Postmortem examinations carried out after the accident showed that many of the passengers were alive when they hit the ground. Of course, unlike the pilots, they had the benefit of the oxygen masks that deploy automatically, and while these only intended to supply oxygen long enough to allow the pilots to bring an aircraft suffering decompression down to a level where breathing is possible without masks, they would have helped.

The Time Line

The details of what happened on that flight are shown by the following time line, where the time in hours and minutes is the elapsed time from departure:

00 hours 00 minutes (09:07 Cyprus time)

Departure from Larnaca for Athens with an estimated flight time of one hour twenty minutes.

00:04

Crew reports problems—cabin altitude warning horn sounds at ten thousand feet, but because the same horn also denotes Takeoff Configuration Warning, crew assume it is a false alert. At fourteen thousand feet, passenger cabin oxygen masks deployment lamp (presumably) illuminates in cockpit.

00:07

"Master Caution" alarm sounds at seventeen thousand feet. Instruments show an apparent problem with the avionics cooling system, caused by the thinness of the circulating air.

The German-born captain and Cypriot first officer spend five or more minutes discussing the problem of the horn with the English maintenance engineer at their base on Cyprus, who says the horn can be silenced by tripping the circuit breaker on a panel behind the captain's seat. The captain leaves his seat, but because of the exertion he collapses before being able to trip the breaker.

The last contact with the aircraft was as it climbed through 28,900 feet.

00:11

Autopilot takes aircraft up to its 34,000-foot cruising height, where it levels out and flies on for one hour toward Kea Island.

01:13

Aircraft overflies Kea VOR at 34,000 feet and continues at that height, ready to turn into the Athens Airport Approach. It duly turns, but as there is no pilot to initiate descent, it stays at 34,000 feet, and the flight director, interpreting it as a missed approach, flies on before executing a roughly 290-degree turn to bring itself back to the Kea beacon.

01:31

Aircraft joins Kea holding pattern, making repeated circuits.

02:17

As the aircraft executes its sixth circuit in the Kea holding pattern, it is intercepted by two Greek F-16 aircraft. They report, "Captain not in his seat; first officer slumped over controls; passenger oxygen masks dangling."

02:42

Pilots of the F-16s see a male entering the aircraft's cockpit, sitting in the captain's seat, and trying to regain control of the plane.

02:43

Left engine flames out due to fuel depletion; aircraft loses height.

02:47

Cockpit voice recorder CVR records two Mayday messages transmitted with a labored voice. They are not received on the ground, as the frequency is still set to that for the departure point, Larnaca.

02:53

> The right engine flames out at an altitude of 7,100 feet.

02:56 (12:03 local time)

> The aircraft crashes into hilly terrain near the village of Grammatikos, about twenty miles northwest of Athens International Airport.

According to early reports, even though the fuel had essentially run out, the flammable brush and grass meant fires smoldered for several hours, making many of the bodies difficult to identify. However, the body of a female flight attendant was found in the cockpit area, and that of a male flight attendant with some general aviation (private pilot) experience was found slumped on the controls.

The medical report suggested that some passengers were alive, but no doubt unconscious, when the aircraft hit the ground. This is somewhat surprising since the passengers' emergency oxygen masks only supply oxygen for a limited time.

The final report by the Greek investigators made the following conclusions.

Direct Causes

1. Nonrecognition that the cabin pressurization mode selector was in the MAN (manual) position during performance of the preflight procedure, "Before Start" checklist, and "After Takeoff" checklist.

2. Nonidentification of the warnings and the reasons for the activation of the warnings (cabin altitude warning horn, passenger oxygen masks deployment indication, indication, "Master Caution") and continuation of the climb.
3. Incapacitation of the flight crew due to hypoxia, resulting in continuation of the flight under the control of the flight management computer and the autopilot, until depletion of the fuel and engine flameout, and subsequent impact of the aircraft with the ground.

Latent Causes
1. The operator's deficiencies in organization, quality management, and safety culture, documented diachronically as findings in numerous audits.
2. The regulatory authority's diachronic inadequate execution of its oversight responsibilities to ensure the safety of operations of the airlines under its supervision. Inadequate responses to findings of deficiencies documented in numerous audits.
3. Inadequate application of crew resource management (CRM) principles by the flight crew.
4. Ineffectiveness and inadequacy of measures taken by the manufacturer in response to the previous pressurization incidents in this particular type of aircraft, both with regard to modifications to aircraft systems as well as guidance to the crews.

Contributing Factors

1. Omission of returning the pressurization mode selector to "Auto" after unscheduled maintenance on the aircraft.
2. Lack of specific procedures on an international basis for cabin crew to address the situation of loss of pressurization, passenger oxygen masks deployment, and continuation of the aircraft's ascent (climb).
3. Ineffectiveness of international aviation authorities in enforcing implementation of corrective action plans after relevant audits.

The investigators essentially said that while the maintenance people contributed to the accident by not setting the cabin pressurization mode to automatic, the pilots should have picked this up in three separate checks, and should have subsequently realized the nature of the problem, if not from the warning horn, then from the deployment of the passenger cabin oxygen masks and the Master Caution alert.

Flight International has said that Helios's lawyers claimed the pilots could not have made such mistakes, despite the nonvolatile memory in the pressurization mode unit having showed the controls were set to "Manual" during the flight.

The attempts by the male flight attendant with some piloting experience, in the presence of a female flight attendant, to save the aircraft were not really part of the inquiry.

It seems they were only able to gain entry into the cockpit using a code very late on, by which time the oxygen they had was possibly running out, and the fuel certainly was. Had they been able to gain access earlier, and had they been able to communicate by radio for advice on how to fly the aircraft, it might have been a somewhat different story.

(It has been argued by some that measures taken since 9/11 to make it impossible to gain access to the flight deck without authorization from the pilots could be counterproductive in such circumstances.)

The report criticized the regulatory authorities, saying this was not the first time such a problem had occurred and that those authorities should have insisted the manufacturer did more to prevent such an error remaining undetected.

Founded in 1999, Helios Airways changed its name to A Jet Aviation Limited in April 2006, while continuing operations with its two remaining Boeing 737-800 aircraft.

In *The Crash Detectives*, Christine Negroni says that a Helios mechanic and three executives facing criminal charges in the accident hired experts to help defend them. According to them, examination of scoring on the back of the selector knob showed it might have been pushed to the off position in the crash.

That would have meant the crash was due to mechanical failure.

Her point is that one can never be sure, though one must wonder about conclusions drawn by those with an interest in the outcome. Even then they only said "might."

Chapter 15
MILITARY ACTION

For the full version of these accounts please see the original all-in-one single volume version of this book.

Korean Airlines Flight 902 Off Course (Kola, Russia, 1978)

Russian military shocked at its vulnerability

> A passenger had noticed that the sun was on the wrong side of the aircraft but apparently thought the pilots must know what they were doing. They were off course and about to be shot down over the Soviet Union.
>
> Korean Airlines Flight 902, April 20, 1978

The Korean Airlines 707, en route from Amsterdam to Anchorage, Alaska, had for some unknown reason deviated from its course soon after reaching Iceland. The sweeping deviation to the right was so gradual that it could not have been made manually, and the likely cause was a drift in the inertial navigation system, or the inputting of erroneous waypoint coordinates.

From the initial size of the blip on their radar, the Russians first thought it would prove to be a harmless Boeing 747, but when the fighter pilot announced it was a civilian 707, they had their doubts, as the same design under the designation RC-135 was used by the Americans for intelligence purposes.

With great reservations, the Russian pilot fired off two missiles, the first of which failed to detonate, while the second exploded in the vicinity of the 707's left wing, damaging the fuselage and killing two passengers. The Korean pilot initiated a rapid descent to a height where the passengers could breathe without their oxygen masks.

In so doing, he entered low cloud and incidentally became invisible to the fighters, which had overshot him. On turning back, they failed to locate him, and, unaccompanied, the pilot flew on for almost an hour, looking for somewhere to land, before finally successfully bringing the aircraft down safely on a frozen lake.

The fact that a possibly hostile aircraft could fly low and undetected over its territory for such a long time came as a great shock to the Russian military. Though it realized there had been no intrigue, it feared the Americans might have learned much from the event and might exploit that newfound loophole for military purposes.

The passengers were quickly returned, and the crew somewhat later.

Korean Airlines Flight 007 Off Course (Sakhalin Island, 1983)

Airline again provokes paranoid Soviet defense forces

> Heads rolled after the incident just described, and the climate was such that all involved would do their utmost to ensure another intruder did not get through.
>
> Korean Airlines Flight 007, September 1, 1983

On September 1, 1983, Korean Airlines Flight KAL007, en route from Alaska to Seoul, had a similar course deviation as that incurred by KAL902 five years earlier. However, this time the

Boeing 747 had already passed over militarily sensitive areas of Eastern Russia and was heading possibly for the even more sensitive area around Vladivostok. The aircraft was eventually shot down by a Russian fighter just off the northern coast of Japan.

All 269 passengers and crew lost their lives.

Though more details of the Russian action became available much later, there has always been some suspicion that the downed flight was not as innocent as claimed. It was the subject of a couple of movies.

The US president finally decided to allow GPS for civilian use, as that would have prevented the airliner getting "lost.".

US Warship Downs Iranian Airliner (Persian Gulf, 1988)

Possibly resulted in Pan Am 747 Lockerbie disaster

A fabulously expensive US warship designed to fight World War III, with a "gung-ho" captain, found itself larking around with Iranian gunboats in Iranian territorial waters, and in the process shot down an Iranian airliner on a scheduled flight.

Iran Air Flight 655 and USS *Vincennes*, July 3, 1988

The "Sea of Lies" article in *Newsweek* (July 12, 1992), still available online today, is one of the best in-depth accounts of what happened, covering the events leading up to the incident, the incident itself, and the cover-up that followed.

It was not so much the USS *Vincennes*'s captain's decision to fire based on mistakes by his crew, but his pursuing Iranian speedboats representing no real threat in order to claim combat experience.

MH17 777 Shot Down by SAM Missile (Ukraine, 2014)

It could have been another airliner

> It was a matter of being in the wrong place at the wrong time, but should they and other more revered airlines have risked being there?
>
> Malaysia Airlines Flight 17, July 17, 2014

Taking the shorter route eastwards from Western Europe, as did more than fifty other airlines per day, the Malaysian Airways 777 was flying over a war zone on the Ukrainian side of the border with Russia.

Ben Sandilands, on his blog, *Plane Talking*, has pointed out that, strictly speaking, airlines should not have allowed their twin-engine aircraft to fly that route, as they would not be able to maintain that altitude should an engine fail. Anyway, the BUK missile that shot down the Malaysian 777 was effective up to an altitude of eighty thousand feet, more than double the height it was at.

Russia was blamed for putting such a weapon in the hands of fighters over the border in the Ukraine, but obviously did not intend for them to shoot down an airliner. Now airlines are more careful about war zones.

Chapter 16
TERRORISM

Air India 747—Deadliest Bomb on a Plane (North Atlantic, 1985)

A second bomb explodes at Tokyo's Narita Airport

> This was the first instance of a jumbo jet being downed by an onboard explosive device.
>
> Air India Flight 182, June 23, 1985

Explosion at Narita Airport

At 06:19 UTC on June 23, 1985, two Japanese baggage handlers were killed, and four others injured at Tokyo's Narita Airport as an item of luggage was being transferred to Air India Flight 301. It had come from Montreal on a CP Air flight. Whoever had set the timer had apparently not realized Japan does not have summertime, in which case the bomb would have gone off when the aircraft was airborne.

Air India Flight 182

One hour later, Air India Flight 182, bound for London from Montreal with 329 people on board, exploded in midair off the west coast of Ireland, and fell from 31,000 feet (9,400 meters) into the sea with no survivors.

Backdrop

In 1983, armed Sikh separatists took over Sikhism's holiest shrine, the Golden Temple complex at Amritsar,

India. From there the separatist leader agitated for a Sikh homeland called Khalistan in the northern Indian state of Punjab.

In early June 1984, Indian prime minister Indira Gandhi ordered an attack by the Indian army on the temple in which the separatist leader and his supporters were killed, together with hundreds or more innocent pilgrims. This not only led to demonstrations around the world but to the assassination of the Indian prime minister by two of her Sikh bodyguards, in turn leading to the 1984 anti-Sikh riots, in which thousands of Sikhs in India were killed.

Earlier, a number of militants wanted by the Indian government had fled abroad, with countries refusing to return them. Many ended up in Canada, and in Vancouver there were demonstrations and firebrand speeches by activist leaders seeking revenge. There was also intimidation of moderates—one of them, a prominent Sikh lawyer, was beaten up by someone with a metal bar in February 1985, and he wrote to the prime minister that April saying he should act before something serious happened.

The Canadian Security Intelligence Service (CSIS), created only a year before, were in fact following a Sikh leader called Parmar, even tailing him on June 4, 1985 to Duncan, on Vancouver Island, where he met Inderjit Singh Reyat, a local Sikh marine mechanic, and another man. They drove to a wood, where the agents lost sight of them. They did hear what sounded like an explosion but could not be sure.

The Investigation

The CVR and FDR for Air India Flight 182 were recovered after two weeks, but all they could show was that the flight had been completely normal. Despite the great depth of the water, some large pieces of wreckage were recovered before severe weather set in and showed that an explosion had occurred in the front luggage bay just aft of the avionics bay.

However, tiny pieces that might have provided clues as to who might have made the explosive device were scattered over a wide area deep under water, unlike at Lockerbie, where by unbelievable luck a key one was found. However, things were different in Tokyo, where the bomb had gone off in a confined space with it even possible to recover fragments embedded in the walls.

On the fragments, the Japanese investigators found the serial number of the Sanyo tuner that held the explosive. It was one in a batch of two thousand that had only been sold in British Columbia. Canada's Mounted Police were eventually able to find the shop in Duncan that had sold it to a Sikh called Reyat!

How Was It Allowed to Happen?

A browbeaten airline check-in clerk, to her everlasting regret, allowed luggage to be booked through without a confirmed booking, the two aircraft were allowed (in those days) to depart with luggage of no-shows, and a case that raised suspicions was not properly checked. Also, the Canadian government had ignored repeated warnings.

Prosecutors hoped bomb maker Reyat would testify against his coconspirators, but he led them on a song and dance, saying at the trials he could not remember, resulting in him being later convicted of perjury. As it was the then policy of the newly created CSIS to erase tapes of intercepts following their translation, it meant evidence against others did not stand up in court.

Witnesses were murdered, threatened, and the suspects walked free.

The official inquiry in 2010 said in part:

A cascading series of errors contributed to the failure of our police and security forces to prevent this atrocity.

The level of error, incompetence, and inattention which took place before the flight was sadly mirrored in many ways for many years, in how authorities, governments, and institutions dealt with the aftermath.

Failed Precursor to 9/11 (Marseille, 1994)

Target was Eiffel Tower or Elysée Palace

> In 1994, French special forces stormed a hijacked Air France airliner that terrorists intended to use for a 9/11-style outrage in Paris. The French authorities claimed it was one of the most successful operations of its kind ever.
>
> Air France Flight 8969, December 24 to 26, 1994

At 11:15 a.m. on December 24, 1994, Air France flight AF8969, an A300 Airbus, was about to depart for Paris from Algiers Airport, with 220 passengers and 12 crew.

Hijacked on The Ground

As Algeria was in a state of civil war, passengers did not think it untoward that four armed men dressed in sharp blue uniforms with Air Algérie insignia claiming to be security agents came on board to make a final passport check before departure. That is until there were shouts of "Allahu Akbar!" ("God is great!") from the four "security men," who, having abandoned their passport checks and stayed inside, shut and locked the doors.

Three of them quickly proceeded to the cockpit, while the fourth kept the passengers at bay by waving a gun at them. For those at the back of the aircraft, it was quite difficult to work out what was going on, and later some even remained unaware that selected passengers had been used as bargaining chips and shot.

Algerian special forces, already on high alert at the airport, as the country was in a state of civil war, came to see what was going on and quickly confirmed the individuals were terrorists. They belonged to the Algerian Armed Islamic Group (AIG).

It being Christmas Eve, many top French officials were away on vacation and, as usual, Prime Minister Balladur was at his Alpine chalet, in Chamonix, where he stayed glued to the phone line for the first day. The French foreign minister and interior minister were in Paris handling the situation, their roles being to deal with the Algerian authorities and set up a team ready to go into action and overcome the hijackers should that prove necessary.

The hijackers' immediate demand had been the release from house arrest of two leaders of the Islamic Salvation Front (FIS), an Algerian organization banned in Algeria. The hijackers negotiated via the pilots with the Algerian interior minister, who had rushed to the airport and was using the radio equipment in the control tower.

After an hour or so the hijackers seemed more intent on going to Paris than seeking the release of the two political leaders. To try and move things along, they shot an Algerian policeman, whom they had identified during the passport checks. He was led away begging not to be killed, as he had a wife and child. His body, still quivering, was dumped outside the aircraft.

With the Algerian authorities still adamant, the hijackers then killed the commercial attaché at the Vietnamese embassy in Algeria, who was the only person on board who was neither Algerian nor French; the poor man, thinking he was being released, went back for his coat.

The Algerian authorities insisted on the release of the elderly, invalids, children, and so on, and by the end of the second day, Christmas Day, the hijackers had released sixty-three in all. Their departure probably made it easier for the terrorists to handle things in the aircraft, where they established a strict and oppressive regime without being rude.

First, they made women and men sit separately and use different toilets. They also ordered the women, including the flight attendants, to cover their faces with whatever material was available, which included cut-up blankets. Then, applying psychological intimidation, the hijackers instituted a regime whereby they would treat the passengers harshly for twenty minutes, allow them to relax for twenty minutes, and then repeat the process. The intention of this "torture," as some described it, was probably to keep the passengers off balance.

The authorities managed to identify the leader of the hijackers and even had his mother brought to the airport to try to persuade him to let the passengers go. This only seemed to provoke him further.

Meanwhile, the French had not been wasting time. Right at the start they put their Special Deployment Unit (National Gendarmes Intervention Group, or GIGN) on standby. This was an elite police unit trained along military lines for intervening in hijacks and hostage situations.

Although they had not been able to get the Algerian authorities to agree to let them help, a team of forty of these elite commandos set off in an A300 Airbus for

Palma de Mallorca, in Spanish territory, some two hundred miles north of Algiers.

Balladur, the French prime minister, had returned to Paris to take overall command, and as the evening of the second day approached, the hijackers, worn down and tired, realized they were getting nowhere slowly. After threatening to blow up the aircraft, they issued an ultimatum. If the boarding ramp was not pulled back and the plane not allowed to take off before 9:30 p.m., they would kill a hostage every half hour.

Announcing that the first to be shot would be Yannick Beugnet, a cook at the French ambassador's residence in Algiers, they brought him to the flight deck and allowed him to plead for his life over the radio. The cook was then shot, and his body thrown onto the tarmac. Balladur was livid at the news, telling the Algerian prime minister they would hold him responsible. He then called the Algerian president, saying he expected to see the imminent arrival of the aircraft on French soil.

Arrival of Aircraft in Marseille

The aircraft took off in the early hours of the next day, December 26, and at 3:30 a.m. landed at Marseille, where the hijackers had been told a refueling stop was necessary. There was an element of truth in this in that much of the fuel initially loaded in Algiers for the flight to Paris had been consumed by the auxiliary power unit (APU), which had been kept running to keep the lights and air-conditioning working.

The Special Deployment Unit had taken off from Majorca in its A300 and followed them to Marseille, touching down at an adjacent military base. In Majorca, the commandos had had time to fully familiarize themselves with the layout of an A300 and prepare. On the ground in Marseille, they went through their routines again.

Meanwhile, the Marseille chief of police was conducting negotiations with the hijackers, the aim being to wear them down further and, if possible, delay any action until dusk, which would be quite early, as it was the middle of winter.

The French had received information that the hijackers intended to blow up the aircraft over Paris, and very likely on a landmark there. Passengers released in Algeria had described how explosives were set up in a way that demolition experts said indicated they would cause the aircraft to explode. This belief was further reinforced by the terrorists' demand for twenty-seven tonnes of fuel, when only ten tonnes would largely suffice to get to Paris. Anyway, the French were determined not to let the aircraft leave Marseille.

At dawn, the hijackers issued an ultimatum, but the negotiators were able not only to extend this but also exploit it by saying some servicing was needed. They sent in commandos in disguise, ostensibly to provide food and water, clean and service the toilets, but in reality, to plant snooping devices, identify who was who and where.

They noted that the doors were neither blocked nor booby-trapped. As the afternoon wore on, with no fuel delivered to the aircraft, the negotiators drew things out by saying that holding a press conference in Marseille would be preferable, as the press was there. They even exploited that by having the hijackers move the passengers toward the back of the aircraft, ostensibly to make more room for the press conference, but in fact to make more room for the commandos and to enable them to separate any hijacker in the cockpit—and possibly in charge—from the others.

As 5:00 p.m. approached, the exhausted hijackers knew things were getting critical for them, and their leader came into the cabin to select a hostage to kill—the youngest member of the cabin crew. However, it seems he was hesitating to put his threat into execution, perhaps out of fear of provoking the French. Instead, in their frustration the hijackers let off some rounds in the direction of the control tower, where they knew the scheming negotiators would be.

The commandos would eventually have moved in anyway, but their firing of shots at the control tower resulted in Prime Minister Balladur giving the head of the special forces carte blanche.

Their plan was to have three teams, who would use boarding ramps to access the doors. Two would creep up from the back, trying to keep out of sight of the hijackers, and open the doors at the back to provide a good escape route for the hostages. The third, led by Major Favier, would have the most difficult role of penetrating the aircraft via the front right door to separate hijackers on the flight deck from their companions.

Despite the commandos having planned and rehearsed the operation so meticulously, the ramp they were standing on proved to be too high to allow them to open fully the right front door they had prized ajar. Then, on quickly pulling it back to allow enough space, they almost left a commando dangling between the fuselage and the ramp. Fortunately, he had a good grip on the door and was able to hang on there until it was opened successfully. They were met with a hail of bullets, with one lucky shot from the hijackers hitting a gendarme's gun, setting off the rounds it contained and knocking him backward down the steps with quite severe injuries.

As hostages evacuated from the rear doors, the commandos progressively overcame the hijackers, though one held on, firing round after round, for almost twenty minutes.

Sharpshooters firing from the control tower were at the beginning unable to get shots in because of the presence of the aircrew.

The first officer then slid out of a broken cockpit window, only to injure himself quite seriously on hitting the ground after dropping from such a height. No hostage was killed—the commandos had flak jackets and the aircrew said the bodies of the hijackers had at times shielded them.

Another reason given for the survival of all the crew was that they had built up a rapport with the hijackers, who could so easily have killed them out of spite.

Favier, the commando leader, suggested it was a matter of mutual respect. Was it the Stockholm syndrome in reverse, in that the hostage-takers began sympathizing with the hostages?

[The term "Stockholm syndrome" comes from a famous case in Stockholm, where hostages kept for several days in a bank ended up empathizing with the hostage takers.]

Bomb under Seat Was Trial Run for Bojinka Plot (Okinawa, 1994)

Bombs were to be placed on eleven US airliners

> Even when closely following people planning a terrorist act, it can be difficult or impossible for the security services to be sure of their intentions, let alone have material that would stand up in court. Here, a chance fire led them to a laptop computer revealing all.
>
> Philippines Airlines Flight 434, December 11, 1994

The massive Boeing 747 bound for Tokyo had stopped at the Cebu Airport, having come from Manila. There, some passengers, including one traveling under a false name who had spent some considerable time in the toilet and then sat for a while in seat 26K, which was not his, had descended.

Most of the 273 passengers boarding at Cebu were Japanese. There was a crew of twenty, including the captain, fifty-seven-year-old Eduardo "Ed" Reyes, Second Officer Jamie Herrera, and Flight Engineer Dexter Commendador. All three were former air force pilots.

Having taken off thirty-eight minutes late due to congestion, the 747 was flying at thirty-three thousand feet and not yet beyond Okinawa when there was an explosion. The autopilot immediately corrected the bank to the right, and since there was no cabin depressurization, there was no need for an emergency descent.

Back in the cabin, eleven passengers were injured, and the one in 26K seemed to be in extremis.

Passengers tried to move away from where the explosion occurred, but flight attendants ordered them to remain seated. Lead economy-class flight attendant Fernando Bayot did move the injured passenger in 27K, who had injuries to his legs, before trying to help the Japanese man in 26K, below whom there was a hole in the cabin floor. He lifted him up, only to find that much of his lower body was missing and had fallen into the cargo hold below. Though the man then expired, Bayot instructed the flight attendants to administer oxygen and make it look as if he were being treated, thus avoiding panic. Eleven passengers were injured, some seriously. After Bayot told him the situation, the captain sent the flight engineer to assess the damage.

Though the autopilot was keeping the aircraft level, input of turns had no effect. The captain was loath to disengage it for fear that the aircraft would enter an irrecoverable bank, but finally they had to risk it, only to find the yoke had no effect either.

With Tokyo two hours away, they decided to make an emergency landing at Naha, on Okinawa, but only managed to make themselves understood after an American took over from the Japanese controllers. Using differential engine thrust, they managed to make the wide turn toward Naha.

Following the first officer's suggestion, they dumped thirty-six tonnes of fuel to reduce landing speed and for there to be less fuel to feed a fire, should one break out.

After a control check—flying the aircraft as if landing to see whether they would have the minimal control necessary—they touched down safely.

Apart from the professionalism of the aircrew, the passengers owed their survival to the fact that the 747 in question was an ex–Scandinavian Airlines version, where row 26 was not above the central fuel tank.

Bojinka Plot to Down Eleven Airliners

The man who had planted the explosive device under seat 26K was Ramzi Yousef, a self-confident operative who had planned the ground-level bombing of the World Trade Center in 1993, leaving underlings to be arrested thanks to discovery of a part with a serial number from the van used.

In Manila, he was planning to kill the pope on his forthcoming visit, down eleven airliners using onboard bombs—Flight 434 was a test for that—and have a man called Murad fly a small plane into the CIA's headquarters.

A couple of weeks after placing the bomb on the Philippine Airlines flight, Yousef, Murad, and another conspirator were preparing bombs in an apartment that was near the papal nuncio's residence and on the route the pope would take. They were relaxed and enjoying soft drinks when Murad went to the sink to wash his hands. Bomb-making chemicals they had been mixing there had not been flushed away.

When water Murad was using splashed on them, they coalesced, starting a fire with acrid smoke that could not be extinguished. Yousef and Murad fled into the street and watched from the other side as the fire services dealt with the fire. Yousef, protecting himself as usual, told

Murad to go back and retrieve the laptop with all their plans.

The local police chief, a woman, thought a fire on the papal route and so near the papal nuncio's residence, where he would be staying, worth investigating. She arrested Murad and declined to release him despite the offer of what was an incredible bribe for someone on her small salary.

Once the encryption was broken, the laptop revealed details of the so-called Bojinka Plot, including flights to be targeted, with even timings for the fuses. That alone could have resulted in some four thousand deaths—more than 9/11! There were even details regarding the planned crash into the CIA headquarters at Langley, Virginia. After painful interrogation, Murad revealed even more details.

US Diplomatic Security Service (DSS)—Yousef

A partial fingerprint of Yousef's was also found. He had once again got away, but a month later he was arrested in Pakistan thanks to shrewd handling of a walk-in at the US embassy by US Diplomatic Security Service (DSS) agents. By not going through prescribed official channels they avoided him being tipped off.

9/11—World Trade Center and Pentagon (USA, 2001)

Protocols for dealing with hijacks turned on their head

> Since there were relatively few passengers on board the fuel-laden early-morning flights, it was the 2,700 people on the ground killed by those aircraft that made the tragedy so terrible.
>
> American Airlines Flight 11, September 11, 2001
> United Airlines Flight 175, September 11, 2001
> American Airlines Flight 77, September 11, 2001
> United Airlines Flight 93, September 11, 2001

Nineteen terrorists hijacked four aircraft almost fully laden with fuel for long transcontinental flights. They intended to fly them into symbolic US buildings. Hijackers on three of the four aircraft succeeded in doing this.

With so many excellent accounts, documentaries, and movies covering the events of 9/11, it would be difficult to add usefully to them here. However, the timeline below, presented in tabular form, is perhaps a useful tool for grasping how the overall situation developed. The operation depended largely on timing and doing the deeds before people, and in particular those on the aircraft, realized what was happening. The outcome could have been even worse had airport congestion not delayed the takeoff of the fourth aircraft, enabling the passengers to learn the hijackers' real intentions.

For unknown reasons, the four hijackers on that last flight, UA93, were rather slow in going into action, despite already being behind time due to the thirty-five-minute delay in taking off. When they did finally hijack the aircraft, passengers and cabin crew inevitably started phoning out, only to learn that their aircraft would probably soon become a flying bomb; if they did nothing, they were goners anyway.

Outline of Events

The FAA's Herndon command center supervises air traffic control for the whole United States. The movie *United 93*, about the passengers in the last of the four aircraft to be hijacked, who rebelled after learning by phone what had happened to the other aircraft, is based to a large extent on what happened there. Its operations director, Ben Sliney, had an overall view of the unfolding situation, which he faced on his first day in the job, having returned to the agency after a period in private law practice. He has very cogently explained how difficult it was to assess what the hijackers were doing and which aircraft had been hijacked.

In an interview with Jeremy Vine on a program broadcast by the UK's BBC Radio 2 promoting the above movie, in which he played himself, Sliney said he heard about the hijacking of an airliner just before attending a meeting. He had not been unduly concerned, as there were well-tried protocols for dealing with hijacks, and hijacks took time to play out and usually ended with no loss of life or serious consequences. Interestingly, the FAA thought September was an odd time of the year for a hijack.

In its role of overseeing air traffic throughout the United States, the FAA's Air Traffic Control System Command Center at Herndon does not communicate with aircraft directly. However, it does receive all the necessary data relating to aircraft movements, weather patterns, delays and problems and special situations, such as military activity and the need to clear airspace for Air Force One, the US president's aircraft. It then gives instructions to ATC centers and other ATC facilities all over the States. It also communicates with North American Aerospace Defense Command (NORAD), responsible for defending North American aerospace.

While the center does not handle individual aircraft, its monitors do show the situation of air traffic throughout the country. If pilots enter the squawk code for a hijack into their transponder, this instantly shows up on its screens, as well as on those of the handling ATC. It is also shown on those at NORAD (North American Aerospace Defense Command), which meant that in the days when the controls for transponders were more primitive, pilots had to be careful not to mistakenly squawk the hijack code and attract the attention of a couple of fighters.

However, none of the four aircraft hijacked that day squawked that code, and as a result the controllers in direct contact were the only ones able to progressively deduct that a given aircraft had been hijacked, from the fact that it was not replying or obeying instructions, was changing course or height unduly, or had its transponder switched off. In some cases, controllers heard snippets of conversation in a foreign language, shouts, or in the case of the first aircraft to be hijacked, an announcement destined for the passengers, but which was transmitted because either one of the pilots keyed the radio mic, or a hijacker did so by mistake, saying, "We have some planes; just stay quiet and you will be okay." In every case the transponders were ultimately switched off, making it difficult to even be sure which aircraft was involved, as the controllers could just see the radar echo, without the flight number and height, on their primary radar.

Thus, the FAA Herndon command center and operations manager, Sliney, only belatedly became aware of the gravity of the situation. Sliney said it was only when he saw CNN coverage of the burning North Tower of the World Trade Center, with most people assuming it had been struck by a light aircraft, that he realized from the size of the hole and the amount of fire that it must have been a big jet, and possibly Flight AA11.

Indeed, it was only when the second aircraft hit the South Tower while everyone was watching the burning North Tower on CNN that the FAA command center could grasp the likely implications of any other hijackings that day.

They exchanged information with NORAD and at times were frustrated that the military liaison man could not seem to put them in the loop. However, in the BBC 2 interview, Sliney expressed sympathy for the military in view of the constraints under which it must have been operating.

Who could order the shooting down of a civilian airliner, and an American one at that?

The first two aircraft struck the twin towers of the World Trade Center in almost perfect fashion from the hijackers' point of view. However, the third aircraft, having taken off from Washington's Dulles International Airport, not far from the Pentagon, was later seen heading for it, with its wings level, as if the pilot knew what he was doing.

Some have said it was a great feat of airmanship for a novice to hit the Pentagon at almost ground level, with the maneuver simulating a perfect landing. However, damage and the effect of the inevitable fire would surely have been much more significant had he been able to bring the aircraft down in the hollow at the center of the five-sided, low-aspect construction, and one wonders whether that was the intention and the piloting was not so wonderful after all.

It is thought that the fourth aircraft was heading for either the White House or, more likely, the massive Capitol Building, perched like a wedding cake at the end of the two-mile National Mall, making it an easy target and as symbolic as the World Trade Center. However, the thirty-five-minute takeoff delay, due to congestion at Newark Airport, coupled with the long time the hijackers for some reason took to take over the aircraft, meant that passengers and cabin crew would learn their likely fate by phone and not be so amenable.

From the phone and other evidence, and as shown in the film *Flight 93*, the passengers on the delayed fourth flight decided to take on the hijackers. They did so and very likely managed to penetrate the cockpit, breaking down the door with a food cart from the galley. Confusion apparently reigned, and the aircraft flew into the ground.

Tracks of the aircraft based on the official 9/11 report.

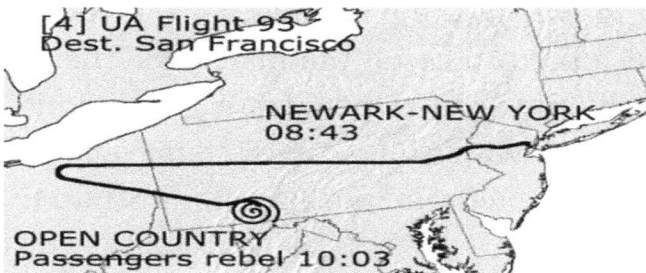

[1] AA Flight 11
Dest. Los Angeles
BOSTON
07:59
NEW YORK
WTC North Tower
08:46

[2] UA Flight 175
Dest. Los Angeles
BOSTON
08:14
NEW YORK
WTC South Tower
09:03

[3] AA Flight 77
Dest. Los Angeles
PENTAGON
09:37
WASHINGTON
08:20

[4] UA Flight 93
Dest. San Francisco
NEWARK-NEW YORK
08:43
OPEN COUNTRY
Passengers rebel 10:03

Some say the hijackers crashed it on purpose. Others have maintained a fighter shot it down just when the heroic passengers had gained control, a story that would not make for pleasant reading. Much material is available on the Internet for anyone interested in exploring the matter further, although as mentioned in Acknowledgments, one can waste a lot of time going down the conspiratorial alley without coming to any definite conclusions.

Hijackers' Modus Operandi

Each of the four hijacker groups included one or more members who had learned how to fly at various flying schools for light aircraft. Their instructors had been surprised that learning how to land did not seem to interest them. Using manuals for the airliners concerned, namely the Boeing 757 and 767, and no doubt PC flight simulation programs, they had acquired the necessary flying skills for their task.

Although some of their number were stopped and searched at the airport security checks, they were allowed to board. It seems bluff played a large part in that they would have a member go into the toilet and come out wearing something harmless made to look like a bomb that could be detonated at any moment if the passengers and cabin crew did not comply with instructions. Should that not suffice, they had other items, including pepper spray, that could be used to subdue or kill.

The fact that there were relatively few passengers on board the aircraft made them easier to control, as it was possible to herd them into the rear of the aircraft, away from the events and the murdered aircrew at the front.

Timeline

Airline Flight Number [sequence]	American Airlines AA 11 [1]	United Airlines UA 175 [2]	American Airlines AA 77 [3]	United Airlines UA 93 [4]	Total Death Toll
Aircraft type	Boeing 767 ER	Boeing 767	Boeing 757	Boeing 757	
Departing	Boston	Boston	Dulles Washington	Newark New York	
Destination	Los Angeles	Los Angeles	Los Angeles	San Francisco	
Passengers	76	51	53	33	213
Crew	11	9	6	7	33
Hijackers	5	5	5	4	19
Total deaths [- hijackers]	92	65	64	44	265 [246]
Actual takeoff	07:59	08:14	08:20	08:42	
Delay in taking off		Approx. 10 min.	Approx. 10 min.	Approx. **35 min.**	
Pilots alerted of danger				09:00 a.m. UA issues system-wide warning of 'cockpit intrusion.' Flight 93 replies 'Confirmed.'	
Hijacked	08:14	08:42	08:52	09:10-09:20	
Airline Flight Number [sequence]	American Airlines AA 11 [1]	United Airlines UA 175 [2]	American Airlines AA 77 [3]	United Airlines UA 93 [4]	Total Death Toll

Hijack suspected	08:20	Immediately	09:05	9:28	
Sounds heard by ATC due to radio mike switch being left on	'We have some planes. Just stay quiet and you will be OK.'			Sounds of scuffling/ Arabic voices	
NORAD informed by FAA	08:40	08:43	09:24?	No available data from NORAD (ongoing exchanges)	
ATC certain	08:25	08:52	08:56	09:32	
Time of impact	08:46	09:03	09:37	10:03 or 10:06 (disputed)	
Level	95th-103rd floors ------------	80th floor -----------	Ground Level --------------	Crash into terrain ----------------	
Location	N. Tower World Trade Center ------------	S. Tower World Trade Center -----------	Pentagon --------------	Open country ----------------	
Effect	Catches fire; tower collapses on itself at 10:29	Catches fire; tower collapses on itself at 09:59	5-storey section collapses	(Passengers confronted hijackers)	
Ground fatalities	**2,793** including woman who died months afterwards due to inhalation of cement, glass, lead and asbestos dust while fleeing the scene. *		125	0	

	Other ATC-related Events			
Between 09:03 and 09:07	**FAA's New York & Boston Regional Centers stop takeoffs and landings**		**NY Port Authority closes Newark Airport**	
09:25	**FAA National Command Center STOPS ALL US TAKEOFFS**			

09:45	FAA orders all 4,500+** aircraft still airborne over the US to land. Orders those that have not yet reached US territory to turn back or land at non-US alternates. ** Under instrument flight rules

* Other than the woman cited, a difficult to determine number of people subsequently became ill or died from the aftereffects of the dust cloud arising from the collapse of the twin towers.

Hijack Protocols

Aircrew, cabin crew, and even passengers had learned that the way to deal with a hijacking was to at least initially comply with the hijackers' demands, and indeed in most cases this had worked well, with the authorities able to wear the hijackers down with endless negotiations on the ground. Normally, special forces would only quickly storm the aircraft if the hijackers commenced systematically murdering the occupants.

The pilots of the last aircraft to be hijacked, United Airlines Flight 93, did receive a warning about cockpit incursion, but unless they were aware that the protocols had changed and the likely consequences, they would have let the hijackers in if they threatened to kill a flight attendant unless they opened the flight deck door.

Nowadays the protocols are different. Cockpit doors are reinforced and are not opened, regardless of any threats made and include a system to that can be set to prevent their being opened even by someone knowing the code.

Passengers are screened more carefully, with flights from abroad required to give details of passengers, and the aircraft turned back or required to land at an isolated airfield if anyone suspicious is on board.

Also, with passengers and pilots aware that compliance with the hijackers' instructions is unlikely to save them, it will be virtually impossible for hijackers to take over aircraft as easily.

The Planners

The events of 9/11 did not represent original thinking in that terrorists had already tried to use an airliner as a flying bomb against the Eiffel Tower. The training of at least one member of each hijacking team to actually fly the aircraft well enough to hit an albeit easy-to-find target was possibly novel.

Probably the biggest issue for the 9/11 planners was how many teams could be prepared before the sheer number risked jeopardizing the entire mission through someone being caught due to bad luck, an error, or loose talk. The choice of early-morning flights, which are less subject to delay and have relatively few people on board, greatly increased the chances of success.

Indeed, it was the terrorists in the delayed aircraft that failed in their mission.

Intelligence Services, CIA, FBI, and NSA

The subsequent inquiry said there were missed opportunities to prevent the outrage which led to soul-searching at the CIA and FBI. However, it did not mention the fact that the National Security Agency was monitoring phone calls two of the hijackers were making from the US to a known Al-Qaeda operations headquarters in the Yemen as they installed themselves, took flying lessons, and purchased flight simulation software.

The NSA did not inform the FBI of this perhaps because of laws, since modified, not allowing them to spy on Americans in the US. Also, and this is the perennial problem for all such agencies, instigating physical surveillance might make the suspects, and in turn possibly very much bigger fish in their network, aware that they are being monitored.

Unintended Consequences of Reinforced Cockpit Doors

In 2015, reinforced cockpit doors that could not be unlocked even with the code prevented the captain of a Germanwings flight regaining entry to the cockpit to stop his suicidal copilot crashing the aircraft and killing all on board.

Liquid Bomb Plot Changed Flying Forever (UK to US, 2006)
Precautions have made flying safer

> The British were closely monitoring a group on the point of blowing up transatlantic airliners using innocuous-looking liquids in drinks bottles. They wanted to delay the arrests until they had enough evidence to stand up in court. The Americans feared delay would result in tragedy and lay them open to accusations of not protecting their citizens.
>
> UK arrests, August 9, 2006

On December 5, 2005, a "person of interest" to the British security services was arriving back at London's Heathrow airport from Pakistan. They could not search him without alerting him, but they could get away with a look inside his checked-in suitcase if done quickly enough. To their disappointment, the only items of any note were a box of batteries and a packet of Tang, a sugar-based powdered soft drink with two orange dyes to make it look like orange juice when mixed with water, made famous through NASA space flights.

The owner of the case was twenty-five-year-old Ahmed Ali, a UK resident with dual British-Pakistani citizenship, who had graduated with a BSc in computer science from City University, London. Unemployed, he was living in a council flat in Walthamstow, East London. From a very young age, he had been meeting people going out to Pakistan and Afghanistan to give aid to those who, with US support, were fighting the Russians and who eventually became the Taliban.

According to a 2008 article in London's *Daily Telegraph*, Ali was already, at age fourteen or fifteen, praising the Taliban and calling for sharia to be introduced alongside British laws.

According to Pakistani surveillance, Ali had met up with a Rashid Rauf, who had fled the UK after possibly murdering his uncle. He not only had high-level links to Al-Qaeda but also bomb-making training. Therefore, anyone associating with such a man needed to be watched, and with Ali back in England, the need was to see in turn with whom he associated.

The closest associate proved to be twenty-six-year-old Tanvir Hussain, an unemployed single man with a child who had also been to university. Then there was Umar Islam, two years older, at twenty-eight. Surveillance continued with not much of note.

Then on July 15, Ali met an unknown individual, and the two of them went to a park, where they lay on the grass facing each other to talk without an observer being able to lip-read, proving they were highly trained professionals. After they separated, the unknown man was followed to High Wycombe, thirty miles outside London, and found to be Assad Sarwar.

A university dropout who had once worked as a postman, Sarwar was living with his parents. He was buying a chemical, hydrogen peroxide, which though quite common and used by hairdressers can also be used to make bombs, such as those used in the London bombings.

Where plots are involved, the security services can spend ages devoting considerable resources—it can take thirty people to follow one individual if three shifts are needed—with nothing to show to a court of justice. Then things can move too quickly for comfort.

The group were found to be visiting a flat of which the security services were unaware. One day someone came out with a bag of rubbish, which they dumped in a bin quite some distance away so it would not be linked to that address. It proved to contain hollowed-out batteries.

Taking one of the greatest risks of the whole operation, the security services planted a bug in the apartment and just managed to get away before anyone returned. This audiovisual bug proved a godsend.

Thanks to it, they were able to see Ali and his associates emptying soft drinks bottles through a hole made in the base and replacing it with a liquid. Listening in, they heard talk about places in the US, such as Miami, Los Angeles, and so on. They also heard Wills being recorded. Ali was followed to an Internet café, where it was found he had downloaded a list of flights to the US leaving around the same time. Their intentions were clear.

Meanwhile the Americans were getting nervous and were not sure the British had everyone in their sights—might someone make a dry run, leading to the loss of an airliner and two or three hundred deaths? The British wanted to wait to have more evidence for the courts, but their hand was forced when the Pakistanis arrested Rauf, very possibly at the indirect instigation of the US.

Everything Changed

From that night on, passengers were no longer allowed to bring liquids or gels with them on board flights, and mothers had to taste milk prepared for their babies. The regulations were later eased, but they remain, as we are all too aware.

The fastidious work by the security services in this case certainly prevented many deaths, though estimates as to the number of aircraft that would have been downed vary widely. It is chilling to think that at least some of the perpetrators intended to bring their wives and children with them. Could it have been to make it easier to bring the materials through security, or could they have wanted their families to share their imagined glory?

The panic ban on liquid in carry-on baggage resulted in many flights from London being canceled.

Shoe Bomber and Underpants Bomber

Individuals acting alone or almost alone can be scary

> Besides the grandiose plots, such as the Bojinka Plot and the Liquid Bomb Plot, a couple of failed ones by individuals have received considerable publicity.
>
> American Airlines Flight 63, December 22, 2001 Northwest Airlines Flight 253, December 25, 2009

Shoe Bomber

Richard Reid was born in England in 1973 with a Jamaican grandfather on his father's side. He was in and out of prison for petty crime, and on the last occasion inside, his father, a habitué of prisons, recommended he convert to Islam for a better life and better food. Upon his release, he attended mosques, including one where the anti-American cleric Abu Hamza al-Masri was holding forth.

He then made trips to Pakistan and underwent training at terrorist camps. On his last trip, he and another British man, Saajid Badat, went on to Afghanistan, where they were given shoe bombs, clunky footwear containing explosive material. On December 5, 2001, he traveled to Brussels, declared his passport lost, and obtained a clean new one from the British embassy.

On December 16, 2001, he traveled to Paris, and the next day he bought a return ticket from there to Antigua via Miami, meaning he did not need documentation for the US. On December 21, 2001, he tried to board the flight, but his disheveled appearance, and the fact that he bought his ticket with cash and had no checked-in baggage, made a security agent suspicious. He missed his flight, with the French police giving him the all-clear to fly the next day, as he did not seem to have anything suspicious on him.

After spending an uncomfortable night in damp conditions, he boarded American Airlines Flight 63 to Miami. Midflight, flight attendant Hermis Moutardier, thinking she smelled a burnt match, saw Reid attempting to light one. He promised to desist, but a few minutes later, as he tried to grasp her, he revealed a shoe in his lap with a fuse leading to it, which he was trying to light.

Several people were needed to overpower Reid, who was six foot three. A disaster had been narrowly averted since the fuse was damp because of the extended wait overnight in humid conditions, and very likely also because of Reid sweating. The other man, Badat, did not board his intended flight but failed to warn the authorities about Reid. Reid never expressed regret and has said he thought that God had not wanted it to happen just then.

Underpants Bomber

The Airbus A330 flight from Amsterdam to Detroit on Christmas Day 2009 had Delta Airlines livery but a Northwest Airlines 253 flight number, as Northwest was a subsidiary. On board were 279 passengers, 8 flight attendants, and 3 pilots. Having taken off at about 08:45 local time, it was due to arrive in Detroit at 11:40 local time.

As the aircraft neared its destination, a young Nigerian man called Abdulmutallab went to the toilet, spending some twenty minutes there before returning to his seat. Complaining of an upset stomach, he snuggled down under a blanket.

Twenty minutes or so before landing, passengers heard popping noises resembling firecrackers, smelled an odor, and saw the Nigerian man's trousers on fire. Jasper Schuringa, from the Netherlands, sitting on the other end of the same row, saw Abdulmutallab shaking with his trousers open and clasping a burning object. Schuringa pulled it from him and tried to extinguish the flames with his hands before jettisoning it. Flight attendants extinguished the fire with a fire extinguisher and blankets, and another passenger removed a partially melted, smoking syringe from the man's hand.

Schuringa grabbed Abdulmutallab and dragged him to the business class area at the front of the plane, where he removed his clothes to check for weapons or other devices. Abdulmutallab was restrained with plastic handcuffs. The virtually undamaged aircraft landed shortly after, and Abdulmutallab was taken into custody and given treatment for his burns.

Like the shoe bomber, he had created a device by mixing pentaerythritol tetranitrate, or PETN, a major ingredient of Semtex belonging to the same chemical family as nitroglycerin, with triacetone triperoxide, or TATP, and other ingredients. Liquid acid injected via a syringe was to be the trigger.

It failed because he had been wearing the underpants for so long, they were soiled and damp.

A Litany of Security Failures

There has hardly ever been a case of so many security failures. The man's father had alerted the US that he posed a danger; the British had flagged him up to the Americans but omitted his surname; the CIA knew about him but did not void his visa because they hoped he would lead them to bigger fish, which reminds one of 9/11, where the NSA were listening in to calls made by one of the hijackers to an Al-Qaeda HQ while undergoing pilot training in the US.

Finally, even without the alerts, the Israeli company, normally so adept at profiling passengers, should have stopped Abdulmutallab boarding—nonsensical routing, ticket bought for cash, and only hand luggage for a long-haul flight.

Chapter 17
"COMPUTERS WORK
IN MYSTERIOUS WAYS"

("THEIR WONDERS TO PERFORM")

Preening A320 Crashes at Local Air Show (Habsheim, 1988)

Playing to the gallery and last-minute alteration of course

> The crash of the innovative Airbus 320 at a tiny air show with passengers on board seemed a bad portent for what was to be—and still is—one of the most successful aircraft ever. Was the pilot responsible? Or was it the computer?
>
> Air France Flight 296, June 26, 1988

C oming from Paris, the brand-new A320 would stop briefly at Basel-Mulhouse Airport to pick up sightseers and then impress spectators at a tiny airshow at an airfield at Habsheim, close to the border with Germany and Switzerland, before going on to show the young passengers France's highest mountain, Mont Blanc, twenty-five minutes' flight time to the south.

Provided the pilots did not sink below the minimum permitted height of 100 feet (30 meters), given in their instructions, and their track kept to that of the 3,300-foot (1,000-meter) paved runway, with an obstacle-free overrun space extending some 650 feet (200 meters) beyond the end, the display location was just acceptable.

However, unbeknown to the pilots, the air show's organizers had placed the spectators facing a grass landing strip used for ultralight aircraft and gliders, set at a forty-degree angle to the paved runway. Besides being only 2,264 feet (690 meters) in length, this grass landing strip ended a mere 200 feet (60 meters) from the edge of a dense forest of young oak and birch trees, with many reaching to a height of 40 feet (12 meters).

A quick glance from above and afar might well have given the impression the closely packed trees represented a different-color field or mere bushes. However, it would seem quite probable that the pilots, with no time to assess the situation, simply presumed the organizers had placed the spectators alongside a landing strip suitable for flying demonstrations, with no immediate obstacles beyond.

Air France management had officially approved the application from the organizers of the air show, but final arrangements were hurried and seemed somewhat haphazard. The company only gave the file with the details of the operation to the pilots just before they left Paris, with no verbal briefing about conditions.

The map of the airfield did not have a key to the symbols used, which might have been obvious had it not been a black-and-white photocopy of a colored map. Air France had previously done flyovers at Habsheim air shows, and it may have seemed to all a routine affair.

Since the two pilots chosen for the jaunt, Captain Michel Asseline, forty-four, and copilot Captain Pierre Mazières, forty-five, were both management captains—always a dangerous proposition—Air France staff perhaps too easily assumed they would be able to responsibly assess the situation for themselves and be able to perform the task without oversight. However, neither of them had experience of giving demonstrations at air shows.

As head of Air France's A320 training division and as one of the people responsible for liaising with the manufacturer over the technical aspects of the introduction of the A320 into Air France's fleet, Asseline had experience of executing the dramatic maneuver he was planning. He would use the ability of the computer to fly closer to the stall limit than a human could normally manage. He told his doubting copilot he had done it twenty times. While true, this would certainly have been over airfields or rather airports with plenty of space and in an A320 probably carrying much less weight in terms of fuel and passengers, if any, and perhaps even more importantly plenty of time to stabilize his approach.

In the mere *five minutes*, it would take them to fly from Basel-Mulhouse airport to Habsheim, they would have to lose height and speed, and lower the flaps and landing gear, before performing a low-level pass at a hundred feet (thirty meters), followed by a dramatic climb-out to impress the spectators. Not really much time even were everything to proceed as expected.

Asseline would reduce the airspeed to just above the minimum needed to maintain horizontal flight and let the computer do the rest—namely, raise the nose very high to keep the aircraft flying parallel to the ground. Of course, to do this he would have to disengage the Alpha floor safety mode, designed to rescue the aircraft from dangerously high angle-of-attack situations, such as might develop in wind shear, and notably in the stunt in question. The Alpha floor safety mode would otherwise apply full takeoff/go-around power via the autothrottle and spoil the party.

Though the computer could be relied on to not let aircraft stall at the minimum airspeed, it would be a risky procedure if there were any obstacles in the aircraft's path, as it would be difficult to climb away at that minimal airspeed, and especially so if the engines were still idling and would therefore take more time to spool up.

It is a tenet of airlines and even the military that pilots making a landing, which this maneuver resembled, conduct a stabilized approach. "Stabilized" means the aircraft should have steadied and be properly lined up, and, as far as possible, be at the right speed well before the runway.

Hurried, last-minute, possibly ill-judged maneuvers are to be avoided. If not stabilized in good time one must abort the landing and go around. The short distance between Basel-Mulhouse, where they were to pick up the passengers, and Habsheim would give the Asseline scant time to descend and stabilize in the best of circumstances. In addition, their unfamiliarity with the area would mean they would be looking for landmarks.

With the sightseers including many children picked up at Basel-Mulhouse Airport on board, and Asseline announcing, "I am going to demonstrate the progress made[1] by French aviation," the jaunt was taking on the trappings of a trip to the circus, which is in fact what it turned out to be.

The subsequent inquiry suggested the presence of the sightseers created a holiday feeling in Captain Asseline.

The A320 turned toward Habsheim with maximum bank and climbed to the thousand-foot altitude authorized by the Basel-Mulhouse Airport control tower. Still at almost a thousand feet, they headed for Habsheim having to refer to a map showing it to the right of the motorway as the "airport" was too small to figure in their navigation system. As a result, they were late in identifying it, leaving them insufficient time to drop down to a hundred feet (thirty meters) and reduce speed to that required for the demonstration.

Asseline suddenly realized that the spectators were placed to view performances along the axis of that grass landing strip, set at a forty-degree angle to that of the paved runway, and some distance to the left. If he maintained his course, he would fly over them, so banked to the right to fly in front of them.

Just when he should have been stabilizing the aircraft at a hundred feet, he lost further height perhaps because aircraft lose some lift when banking. Adding to its vulnerability was the fact that the engines were throttled back to idle so Asseline could get the airspeed down to that minimum flyable airspeed in time for the computer to show off by pushing the nose up at the sharpest possible angle without stalling.

The aircraft did just as it was expected to do, ending up with its nose pointing upward at a maximum of fifteen degrees and with its trajectory virtually horizontal over the grass landing strip.

This would not have been disastrous had the pilots had started the maneuver too low. The dangling main wheels were just thirty feet (ten meters), instead of a hundred feet (thirty meters), above the grass strip.

Some have suggested that having the nose so high up and the tail so low made the pilots feel they were higher than they were. The small scale of the airfield might also have deceived a captain used to runways four times as long and control towers three times as high. Others contest this.

Aircraft sinks into Trees

Moments earlier Mazières had warned Asseline about electricity pylons carrying power lines almost two miles (three kilometers) ahead, and the captain told him not to worry, as he too had seen them. What neither of them realized was that the dark-green patch immediately ahead was a forest with trees so densely packed together that they did not stand out when viewed from above from a distance. As mentioned, some were forty feet (thirteen meters) high.

With the trees dead ahead and as high, if not higher, than they were (in the nose-up cockpit), Mazières was the first to see the danger. He shouted, "Go around!" They applied maximum power, expecting to climb away. However, the aircraft was performing at the corner of its flight envelope, and furthermore having had to lose height with the engines throttled back, it had neither quickly available engine power nor any airspeed margin.

Unlike internal combustion engines on motor vehicles, Jet engines do not instantly give extra power, especially when idling, as indeed these were. This meant the engines would take six, if not eight, seconds just to spool up and begin truly accelerating the aircraft. Had the pilots properly stabilized their approach in a timely manner, the engines would have been at an intermediate power setting and spooled up much more quickly.

If an aircraft is flying normally well above its stalling speed, simply pulling back on the sidestick or control column will make it rise almost immediately. However, here the computer had been "told" to fly at a speed so close to stalling speed its nose was already pitched as high up as it could be just to stay level. Even were the computers to allow the pilots to push the nose up much further, which is unlikely, the aircraft would have doubtless stalled. In addition, that nose-up attitude with the wheels down would already have been producing considerable drag and preventing it from gaining forward airspeed.

One video shows the preening Air France A320 approach and pass in front of the camera. Then, just above the ground, it continues, preening even more to try to maintain its height.

Heading straight for the trees, it must surely heave itself up, but its resources seem to fail it, even though the audio on the video shows the engines were finally spooling up.

As if making a perfect landing, the A320's rear underside brushes the trees, with it still seeming possible it might lift off. It then sinks into the foliage like a drowning swimmer engulfed by waves. A few moments later a dense cloud of smoke billows up from a point slightly farther on. Some spectators wail. A woman cries, "My God!" ("Mon Dieu!")

The two airfield fire appliances, and an ambulance with a doctor who was attending the show, rushed to the scene. Appliances from local fire departments tried to join them, but the larger vehicles were unable to get through the closely spaced trees.

Most Occupants Survive

As the last of the mobile occupants, some with smoldering clothes, made it through the forward exit, the flight attendant there called out to check whether there was anyone left. She got no reply, since the three remaining had already been overcome by smoke inhalation. Exiting at the rear had gone more smoothly, apparently in part because a flight attendant there had experienced an evacuation.

Amazingly, 133 of the 136 people on board managed to escape before fire consumed the entire aircraft, except for the tail and part of a wing.

The passengers owed their relative good fortune to their lack of hand luggage (a point to remember) and the fact that many were young, physically able first-time flyers who had noted the location of the exits during the preflight briefing. Unfortunately, this meant some would not know how to release their seat belt buckle (another point to remember, as they differ from those in cars).

The three that perished were a handicapped boy, a young girl, who had been unable to undo her seat belt, perhaps because she had not been able to do it immediately and people behind had pushed her seatback forward, trapping her against the belt, and a courageous woman who came back to help her.

A female flight attendant helping people exit from the front apparently went back into the cabin to check there was no one left. Not being able to see because of the smoke, she called out and got no reply; perhaps the three were already unconscious due to smoke inhalation.

Thirty-four passengers required hospital treatment for burns and injuries. In addition to suffering from shock and smoke inhalation, the two pilots were briefly hospitalized for minor injuries to the head and collarbone.

TV news bulletins around the world replayed and replayed the dramatic footage of the crash, much to the chagrin of the aircraft's manufacturer (Airbus Industries) and Air France, who had only taken delivery of the aircraft some three days earlier.

The media, and particularly competitors, made much ado about the crash of this innovative aircraft, representing the new so-called fly-by-wire technology, which, thanks to computers, was supposed to enable aircraft to fly more safely. Some people, particularly in America, mocked Airbus, saying it seemed its computer made a perfect landing—on trees.

With this very public loss of their new-generation aircraft, the manufacturer and Air France went into a panic. Many prospective orders were at stake, as was the reputation of Airbus Industries, a consortium of French, German, British, Spanish, and West German companies. For the French it was considered, no doubt justifiably, an affair of state, as it threatened France's budding aircraft industry at a delicate moment.

Aftermath

For a crash where "only" three people died and "merely" thirty-four were injured enough to require hospitalization, a surprising amount of controversy and bitterness ensued for more than a decade, even though investigators recovered the black boxes intact, had the benefit of the pilots being able to explain their actions, and there being several video recordings (some with audio). Nobody trusted anybody.

The various parties—Captain Asseline, the survivors and the injured, Air France, Airbus Industries, and even the French government—fought legal battles and exchanged insults.

An exasperated Air France official was reported as saying, with more than a grain of truth[2], something like, "There would have been less trouble had the people died."

There were accusations that officials had tampered with the black boxes. Air France sidelined as unfit for duty a pilot who came out in support of Captain Asseline. The man in question thereafter remained an implacable foe of the airline and the aviation authorities. He has had no end of trouble ever since on account of his comments and the critical books he wrote, even accusing a cabinet minister of being involved in the alleged tampering of the digital flight data recorder (DFDR) and cockpit voice recorder (CVR) tapes. Reduced almost to the state of a beggar, he pursued the fight on the Internet to keep life and soul together.

As is the case in so many dramatic events—even President Kennedy's assassination—securing the "crime scene" and evidence is not usually uppermost in people's minds at the time. In the rush to analyze the CVR and DFDR tapes, those involved were casual in their handling of those valuable items of evidence. Then, when a judge later ordered their surrender to him, they were not immediately available, leading to increased suspicion that the authorities had been in the process of doctoring them.

Captain Asseline first maintained that the accident had occurred because the engines failed to spool up. Then on seeing video showing how extremely low he was, he suggested the barometric altimeter might have been giving the wrong reading, because of a bug in the software. He also said he pulled the throttles back for a moment when the engines did not respond, as from his experience he knew that was the way to reset the system, but there was no indication of that.

The subsequent inquiry laid the blame for the disaster largely on Captain Asseline but also criticized Air France for its casual approach to the whole operation. His pilot's license was revoked, and Air France dismissed him while retaining the services of Mazières.

Asseline then wrote a book called *Le Pilote—Est-il coupable?* (*The Pilot—Is He Guilty?*), and for years contested the official report.

An Affair of State

It was an affair of state whatever way one looked at it. Most of those claiming there was a cover-up admit that if there was one, the government officials involved did so not for personal gain but with the best of motives.

Regardless of whether any credence can be given to the conspiracy theories, Asseline's envisaged maneuver, which Mazières questioned at the time, was a reckless act over a tiny airfield. Furthermore, Asseline was literally playing to the gallery, even making an additional announcement in perfect German for those of his sightseeing passengers unable to understand French. His statement that he was going to demonstrate the evolution of French aviation was almost the language of a stunt or test pilot, and not that of an airline pilot.

In addition, at Basel-Mulhouse Airport he had been taking part in a press conference rather than concentrating on the operation in hand. One can understand how difficult it would have been in that frame of mind for him to perform his stunt away from the spectators. Apart from the rashness of undertaking such a maneuver at an unfamiliar site with an almost full load of passengers, another fault would seem to be that Asseline took the Air France regulations regarding the hundred-foot fly-past height in a landing configuration—in other words, with landing gear and flaps lowered—too literally.

The hundred-foot minimum height was surely set for large, flat, open areas, such as major airfields or airports.

Asseline would no doubt have easily missed the trees had he aimed to fly at that hundred feet plus thirty-five feet or say fifty feet to allow for obstacles in the general area. This would no doubt have been so, regardless of whether, as he later claimed, his altimeter misled him, his engines had not spooled up as fast[3] as claimed by the investigators, and the aircraft did not lift when he thought it should have done. He should have maintained a greater safety margin and have been prepared for, say, a bird strike affecting an engine. Anyway, there was just not enough time to get the aircraft stabilized.

While Air France management surely had much for which to answer, they were presumably expecting their senior pilot to perform a simple fly past, not a stunt.

Anyway, the captaincy of a ship or aircraft is associated with the concept of command responsibility. Regardless of the poor decisions made by others, the captain should exercise good judgment.

Afterthought—and a Lesson

As said, the passengers were mostly youngish adults or nimble youngsters, with no luggage. Even so, it was it was a very close-run thing. Had the passenger profile been typical of one of today's commercial flights, with more elderly passengers and many collecting their luggage, the tragedy would have been far greater.

Even were Asseline right regarding some aspects—a big if—the rushed maneuvering for a stunt in a constricted area, with no time to stabilize the aircraft was a recipe for disaster.

Not having the spectators positioned beside the main paved runway and Asseline not sticking to the original plan to fly along it precipitated the disaster.

This stunt resembled coming in to land, in which case a pilot, on being told to change runways at the very last instant, would execute a go-around.

Showmanship took precedence over airmanship, as in a far greater disaster where a sightseeing DC-10 flight to the South Pole flew into Mt. Erebus (see Chapter 13).

---

[1] He used the French word "continuité," which is difficult to translate. "The march of ..."?

[2] Proved right in the case of the Concorde crash, where everyone died, and claims were settled easily.

[3] The manufacturer of the engines subsequently improved their response time.

Indian Airlines A320 in Wrong Descent Mode (Bangalore, 1990)

Another A320 crash; aircraft too sophisticated?

> Just as Airbus seemed to be leaving the bad publicity of the Habsheim fiasco behind it, there was another Airbus A320 crash.
>
> Indian Airlines Flight 605, February 14, 1990

The Indian Airlines A320 Airbus had taken off from Bombay (Mumbai) with 146 people on board, including two captains in the cockpit. Both captains were experienced but had comparatively few flying hours on the A320, which with its sophisticated computer systems differed considerably from the aircraft they had previously flown, notably turboprops and 737s.

On the final part of the flight into Bangalore, in Southern India, the route-checking captain in the right-hand seat was the pilot flying (PF). This was a strange state of affairs, as the check captain had only flown about sixty-eight hours in the A320 and was not certified by Airbus Industries to be a check captain on the A320.

Furthermore, the Indian civil aviation authorities had instructed the airline that the captain in question be positively monitored with regard to matters such as the sophisticated flight management guidance system (FMGS) on the A320. Not only that, the people instructing him on the A320 had observed "numerous small errors and omissions" regarding the use of the FMGS and operation of the power controls.

At one point the captain undergoing the check asked whether the check captain flying the aircraft realized they were in the OIDM mode and suggested they switch to the heading vertical speed mode. The suggestion was apparently ignored.

Making its final approach to Bangalore with its landing gear already lowered, the A320 was descending, but as it descended it started sinking rapidly and was soon below the intended glide path, with its speed less than it should have been for an approach. Although it was obvious they were not going to make the runway, the pilots took no action, despite two sink rate warnings and four altitude alerts.

Only when they were at 140 feet, still sinking rapidly, and with the computer pushing the nose up to a high angle of attack to compensate for the minimal airspeed, did the pilot nonflying (PNF) shout, "Hey, we're going down!" and push the throttle levers for a TOGA (takeoff/go-around). In fact, the Alpha floor safety mode (disabled at the Habsheim air show) ensured the computer was already spooling up the engines.

Even with the engines speeding up faster than certified, and perhaps faster due to improvements made in the light of the Habsheim disaster, the high sink rate combined with excessively low airspeed meant saving the situation would prove impossible in the hundred or so feet available.

With the nose pointing upward, but less than it would had the computer not prevented the aircraft from going into a stall when the pilots pulled their sidesticks back fully, the aircraft came down hard on a golf course over a half kilometer from the runway. After bouncing and forcing its way through some small trees, it skidded over a green. Slowing more but not enough to prevent the embankment around the course shearing off the engines, the aircraft finally ended its headlong charge just before the airport's perimeter wall and caught fire.

Despite the proximity of the airport, the fire service took more than twenty minutes to reach the scene. This was due to the locking of a gate for security reasons, a bad airport road, and lack of a radio link with the control tower. By the time the fire service arrived, it could do nothing except help those who had already escaped. At Habsheim almost everyone on board escaped, even though the A320 had caught fire immediately. This was largely due to them being able to save themselves thanks to the soft landing.

At Bangalore 54 people out of 146 survived. Many were seriously injured. Both pilots perished.

The inquiry found that, contrary to instructions in the operating manual, the aircraft had been descending in open/idle descent mode (OIDM), with too low an airspeed for an approach. It should have been in the heading/vertical speed mode so that the flight director kept the aircraft pointing in the desired direction and, most importantly, controlled the rate of descent, not letting dangerously high rates of descent develop.

Thus, once again it seemed an A320 had crashed because a senior pilot had not used the sophisticated systems wisely and appropriately. Some say the aircraft was too sophisticated for Indian Airlines at the time.

Recriminations

After the crash, the Indian government claimed Airbus was undermining the reputation of Indian Airlines' pilots and said the check captain was an excellent pilot, even though he was not certified by Airbus to be a check captain testing other pilots.

A French newspaper countered by claiming that C. A. Fernandez, the pilot being checked out, had performed badly in stress situations, had been referred for extended basic training in India, and had not been certified as passing. As mentioned, the check captain flying the aircraft had been found wanting by Indian government officials during tests.

Despite this early scare and spat, which led to the temporary grounding of the airline's A320s, the company has since purchased or leased many A320s.

In-flight Upset of Qantas QF72 A330 (off North Australia, 2008)

Passengers with seat belts unfastened hit ceiling panels

> Though computers generally maneuver aircraft better than humans, something can go terribly wrong when they are fed the wrong information.
>
> Qantas Flight 72, October 7, 2008

One can walk nonchalantly down a street for years until one day one is mugged by a hooded man with a gun. Although you may come out of it unscathed you have to take time off work to recover, and whenever you walk down that street you are anxious and hyper alert. This can happen to pilots who for some reason find their computerized aircraft behaving wildly and seeming to do mad things.

As in the case of the Qantas Bangkok overrun, the Australian Air Transport Safety Bureau (ATSB) has produced very comprehensive reports, namely a fact-giving interim report and a final report on the incident we now describe.

As the nub of the reports is technical, namely the performance of the air data inertial reference unit (ADIRU), and the way the computers were programmed rather than human actions, it is really for techies wanting to know how fly-by-wire aircraft work or those who think it might have some relevance to the Air France A330 crash described next.

In the Passenger Cabins

The Qantas Airbus A330, with 303 passengers, 9 cabin crew and 3 flight crew on board, had taken off from Singapore for Perth on October 7, 2008, at 09:32 local time. It was a regular scheduled flight, with flight number QF72.

Having completed almost two-thirds of their journey and with the aircraft cruising at thirty-seven thousand feet, the passengers were relaxing after their meal, with some on their feet to visit the toilet, when the aircraft suddenly pitched slightly downward before pitching nose-down even more. After the aircraft leveled out and climbed to regain height, the same thing happened again, except that the upset was less violent.

The first upset was particularly brutal; passengers were thrown about, with one woman hitting the fascia above her so hard that it left a dent, before falling back with a bleeding head wound. Most of the injured were those who had left their seat belts unbuckled. A few whose seat belts were loosely attached, and often near the limit of their extension, claimed they became unclasped as they were thrown upward—it seems the clasp got snagged under the arm rest. Those standing were injured, as were the two in the toilet—one seriously, the other less so.

Altogether, one member of the cabin crew and 11 passengers suffered serious injuries. Eight members of the cabin crew and 95 passengers received minor injuries, leaving 200 persons (3 crew and 197 passengers) relatively unscathed, though the roller-coaster experience must have been quite traumatic. As these were the officially reported figures, they may not give the full picture, as others could have been treated privately.

On the Flight Deck

At 12:40:28, and a couple of minutes before the first upset, the autopilot disconnected. There followed a series of warnings that this or that system had failed.

At 12:42:27, and with the pilots having had to take control while still trying to evaluate the confusing situation, the nose of the aircraft pitched downward without any such input command from the pilots. The maximum pitch-down angle was about 8.4 degrees, with the aircraft dropping 650 feet. The crew brought the aircraft back to its cruising height of 37,000 feet, all the time trying to deal with the cascade of failure messages. At 12:45:08 the aircraft made an uncommanded pitch down again. However, this second time the pitch-down angle only attained about 3.5 degrees, with the drop in height less too, at just 400 feet.

The aircrew made a "Pan, Pan, Pan" call, used instead of the well-known Mayday call to signify difficulties rather than a full emergency, and diverted to Learmonth, a backup Australian Air Force base also used by civilian aircraft. When informed by the cabin crew of the gravity of some of the injuries, the pilots made a Mayday call.

Because they were unable to enter a GPS approach into the flight management computer, they made a straight-in visual approach from about fifteen nautical miles, acquiring the precision approach path indicator (PAPI) at about ten nautical miles. They touched down safely at Learmonth at 13:50, with the passengers somewhat apprehensive due to the time taken making orbits before landing.

The Investigation

Though there was much information available from the pilots, the digital flight data recorder (DFDR), the cockpit voice recorder (CVR), the quick access data recorder (QAR), the onboard fault-monitoring systems, and data stored in the various units, it was difficult to determine every detail of what happened and why. Adding to the problem is that it was not quite possible to say why the number one ADIRU seemed to have malfunctioned in the way it did, with the investigations even looking at possible extraneous causes, such as special military radio transmissions. Another aspect was that how the computers react to the—possibly false—data they receive from a failed ADIRU depends on how Airbus programmed them.

To see the great lengths to which the investigators have already gone and to learn much about the A330 fly-by-wire control systems, the author suggests the reader download the actual preliminary report, which, as mentioned, is more for the technically minded. As it gives the facts and details of the work done without conclusions, one cannot sum it up, and to do so would risk distortion.

Other Incidents

Virtually any device can fail, and this is why essential ones, such as ADIRUs, are in triplicate, so that the computers can identify the faulty one as the odd one out. The report said the manufacturer in question stated the mean time between failures (MTBF) for the ADIRU model used on the aircraft in question was about 17,500 flight hours. The chance of two failing together would therefore be minimal. Even if they did, that should not affect the flight controls in such as way. Also, Airbus has apparently stated it knows of no such case where the ailerons have been affected, though it seems this aspect was a matter of programming and a rare data input combination.

The ATSB investigated an in-flight upset occurrence related to an ADIRU failure on a Boeing 777-200 aircraft, which occurred 240 kilometers northwest of Perth on August 1, 2005. The ADIRU on that aircraft was made by a different manufacturer and of a different type to that on QF72. Further details of that investigation can be found on the ATSB website.

The ATSB investigated other incidents where the ADIRUs had problems on Airbus A330s, with one occurring geographically rather near and the other somewhat less near the location where this upset happened, leading to speculation that there might be some other factor, such as electromagnetic waves, at play. However, this is thought to be most unlikely.

The ATSB's final report, dated December 19, 2011, attributed the incident to the combination of a design limitation in the flight control primary computer (FCPC) software of the Airbus A330/A340 and a failure mode affecting one of the aircraft's three ADIRUs. This meant that, in a very rare and specific situation, multiple spikes in angle of attack (AOA) data from one of the ADIRUs occurring more than 1.2 seconds apart (that is, longer than the system would retain historic data on the assumption a spike was abnormal) could result in the FCPC commanding the aircraft to pitch down.

Lawyers representing relatives of victims of the Air France 447 crash (see next narrative) attempted to draw parallels with this incident. However, in that case problems with the pitot probes seem to have been a factor, not mentioned at all in this case.

The Pilot's Memories

Almost ten years after this event the *Sydney Morning Herald* published a sober article based on an interview with the just retired Qantas captain who had experienced this traumatic event.

It was picked up by the *Daily Mail* in much more dramatic terms: "It went psycho: Qantas pilot reveals horror moment computers on flight QF72 *broke down*, sending the aircraft nosediving towards the Indian Ocean with 303 passengers on board."

Details had been public knowledge for many years; however, seeing it through the pilot's eyes is very illuminating and adds a valuable perspective.

AF447 Pilots Turned Glitch into Disaster (South Atlantic, 2009)

If only the pilot flying had done nothing—not climbed

> Without being able to get into the head of the pilot flying, one cannot know precisely why he did what he did. However, there were many human contributory factors.
>
> Air France Flight 447, June 1, 2009

The arrivals boards at Paris's Charles de Gaulle Airport indicated Air France Flight 447 from Rio de Janeiro as "Delayed," but with the delay becoming interminable it became obvious that something was seriously wrong. Finally, the airline had to admit the aircraft with 216 passengers and 12 crew had disappeared between Brazil and Africa.

With no Mayday call, and the Airbus A330 lost in an area not covered by radar, the only real clue as to what had happened was a short stream of cryptic ACARS maintenance messages sent from it by satellite to Air France in Paris. These showed the computers had switched to alternate law meaning the protections preventing the pilots flying outside the safe operating envelope were disabled.

A few days later the Brazilians began recovering small amounts of wreckage, including the vertical stabilizer (tail fin), from the South Atlantic Ocean surface. They also retrieved some fifty bodies, including that of the captain.

A French submarine and vessels trawling with sideways-scanning detectors began searching for the locating signal of the digital flight data recorder (DFDR) and cockpit voice recorder (CVR) expecting to find them.

However, they were unsuccessful even though they continued until the batteries in the locators would have run down a month later.

It was claimed this search was unsuccessful because the water was almost two and half miles (four kilometers) deep and the ocean floor very uneven in places.

Neither the wreckage nor the bodies showed any traces of explosives, so a bomb was ruled out. The aircraft had clearly hit the water with considerable force, but with so little evidence the investigation was in a limbo. Speculation was rife. Did the A330 have some inherent defect?

Two years later, when the search was about to be abandoned, the organizers sought the help of US experts using mathematical probability theories to analyze searches where the object has initially been missed. Using their input, searchers rescanned areas where the wreckage might have been and soon found it thirteen thousand feet (four thousand meters) below the surface of the ocean.

The cockpit voice and flight data recorders were recovered intact, and to Airbus's relief revealed there was nothing intrinsically wrong with the aircraft. Though only revealed much later in the course of the judicial inquiry, the CVR had recorded the captain telling the junior first officer he had only had an hour's sleep the night prior to the flight and admitting it was "not enough."

Recap of Technical Terms

"**Normal law**" simply refers to the usual flying mode where the computers controlling the aircraft are receiving reliable data and fly it optimally with "protections" preventing the pilots doing something stupid such as stalling it.

"**Alternate law**" refers to the mode where the computers controlling (flying) the aircraft, having determined that the data, such as airspeed, they are receiving must be unreliable, switch to a simplified operating law, where many of the protections, such as preventing the pilot stalling the aircraft or doing something that could otherwise endanger it, are suspended. On switching to alternate law, autopilot and autothrust disengage, and control is passed to the pilots, who are alerted by a "cavalry charge" audible warning.

"**Pitch**" is the geometric attitude of the aircraft relative to the earth's surface in the longitudinal plane. (Degree of bank is the attitude in the lateral plane.)

The "**angle of attack**," called "**Alpha**" or "**α**" by Airbus, is the angle of the airflow striking the wing. If the aircraft is cruising normally at an appropriate speed, it is often not so very different from the pitch. However, if the aircraft is sinking, say in a stall, where the wings are not providing enough lift to keep it up, the pitch can, say, be five degrees and the angle of attack (the angle of the airflow to the wings) perhaps forty degrees as the aircraft "flops" downward.

The "**flight director**" (FD) bars on the primary flight display (PFD) show what the flight management computer (FMC) thinks the pilot and/or the autopilot should do, but in the absence of valid airspeed data may just try to keep vertical g-forces constant, even when climbing or descending, and are not a valid guide when the aircraft is dropping like a brick in a stall and not actually "flying." They possibly indicated the pilots should climb to cruising height. Usually, the pilots tell the FMC what they intend—for example, at what heights they want to fly at various stages of the flight and the waypoints they want to pass over, and so on.

The "**electronic centralized aircraft monitor**" (ECAM) is a screen indicating, detailing problems, faults, and advising on the action to take.

The Pilots

The eleven hours' duration of the flight back to Paris meant there were three pilots so that they could take turns to rest.

1. **Marc Dubois**, the fifty-eight-year-old captain with approximately 10,988 flying hours of which 1,700 had been on the Airbus A330. He had made 16 south America rotations;

2. Thirty-seven-year-old **David Robert**, the most senior of the two first officers with 6,547 flying hours and 4,479 hours on the A330, including South America rotations.
A graduate of Frances elite ENAC (aviation college), he had been elevated to a management position and was making the trip to keep his pilot's license current. Talking to the captain in Robert's absence the junior first officer referred to him as "he" rather than by his first name suggesting he was viewed as an outsider, perhaps being part of the elite;

3. Thirty-two-year-old junior First Officer **Pierre Bonin** with 2,900 hours and only 807 on the A330 and rated for it six months earlier. He had only made five A330/A340 South America rotations.

Though the aircraft took off three hours six minutes before the crash, the cockpit voice recording starts about two hours before it was deactivated by the impact with the sea. This was because to comply with pilots' unions' insistence that the cockpit voice recorder not divulge private conversations that could be exploited by management this one worked on a two-hour loop, meaning the pilots could talk freely mid-flight on the assumption what was said would be overwritten before arrival in Paris.

Time Line

–02:00:51 Recording starts (Two hours fifty-one seconds before disengagement of autopilot)

Captain Marc Dubois and the junior first officer, Pierre-Cédric Bonin, are alone on the flight deck. Senior First Officer David Robert is resting in the rest station, just behind the cockpit. [We have omitted what is on this early part of the CVR except for the following exchange where the captain says they would not change course to avoid the cumulonimbus clouds (storms) ahead and suggests Bonin, the junior first officer, must be tired.]

–01:55:05 Captain:

We're not going to let some cu-nimbies (cumulonimbus) mess us around.

The French is more vulgar, but our translation conveys the intended meaning.

–01:11:58 Captain suggests junior FO gets some rest:

Try maybe to sleep twenty minutes when he [the senior FO] comes back or before if you want.

Junior FO:

Okay, that's kind. For the moment, I don't feel like it, but if I do feel like it, I will.

Captain:

It'll be a lot for you.

The captain was obviously concerned about the junior FO getting some rest, but it seems odd that the senior FO is allotted proper rest time in the rest station and not the junior FO. When the captain said, "It'll be a lot for you", he would seem to have been thinking of the total flight time of some eleven hours, not to mention the time on duty before takeoff.

−00:18:07 Captain comments on weather conditions ahead:

It's going to be turbulent [bumpy] when I go for my rest

−00:14:08 Captain notes it is time to wake up the senior FO:

Well, right, we just have to wake him up. That's all, eh?

−00:13:59
Sound of high/low cabin chime (−00:13:55) plus there's a noise like a knock on the partition of the rest station

−00:13:49 Captain asks junior FO about who is landing the aircraft:

Er, who's doing the landing? Is it you? Well, right, he's going to take my place.

The junior FO does not reply.

−00:13:45 Captain confirms FO is a PL [fully licensed pilot], plus there's a change in the background noise:

You're a PL, aren't you?

−00:13:44 Junior FO replies in affirmative:

Yeah.

It was quite logical for the junior FO to perform the landing on their return to Paris, as the senior FO had done so on the way out to maintain his currency and keep his license valid while working in management. However, it seems strange the captain is questioning Bonin's qualifications, something he should have noted prior to departure, and even before the outbound flight.

–00:11:36 to –00:11:34 Private conversation

The BEA has omitted this exchange considering it to be of a private nature. However, one wonders whether it was not just the type of conversation that might have thrown useful light on Bonin's feelings concerning Robert.

–00:11:06 Captain colloquially emphasizes his stint is over— sound chair being adjusted:

That's it.

–00:10:39
[Sound of cockpit door opening.]

–00:10:33 Captain to senior FO:

Okay?

–00:10:29 Junior FO to senior FO:

Did you sleep?

–00:10:27 Senior FO replies:

So-so.

–00:10:21 Captain:

You didn't sleep, then.

–00:10:18 Junior FO answers for senior FO:

He, he said so-so. . . so-so.

–0:09:57 Captain announces he is going for his rest:

Well, I'm out of here. ["I'm scarpering" is a more approximate translation, since the French is very colloquial.]

–00:09:46 Senior FO replies to junior FO's comment:

I… I was dozing in fact.

Senior FO asks junior FO whether he is okay.

–0:09:29 Junior FO replies:

Okay.

–0:09:32 Junior FO briefs senior FO on situation in presence of captain

Well, the little bit of turbulence that you just saw we should find the same ahead. We're in the cloud layer. Unfortunately, we can't climb much for the moment because the temperature is falling more slowly than forecast. So, what we have is some REC MAX [recommended maximum height given by computer for the conditions].

–0:08:34 Captain tells junior FO which frequencies to use

Er, sixty-six, forty-nine, fifty-five, sixty-five, and after it's sixty-five, thirty-five.

–00:08:19

[Noises in cockpit. Captain leaving.]

–01:08:05 to –00:06:28 The FOs discuss diversion airports available

–0:06:21 Junior FO:

The intertropical convergence there. Well, we're in it between SALPU and TASIL.

–0:04:10 Junior FO:

We'll call them in the back to tell them anyway because

. . .

–0:04:00 Junior FO talks to cabin crew

Yes, it's in front. Tell me in two minutes. There we ought to be in an area where it will start moving about a bit more than now. You'll have to watch out there.

–00:03:52 to 00:03:46 Dialog between senior cabin crew member probably in the front cabin and junior FO:

All right, are we to sit down?

Well, I think that it might be a good idea to tell your...

Yeah, okay. I'll call the back (flight attendants at the back); thanks a lot.

Thanks. I'll call you when we're out of it.

–00:03:04 Junior FO:

See, we're really on the edge of the layer *[and under the squall]*.

–00:02:02 Senior FO:

Don't you, maybe want to go to the left a bit?

–00:01:58 Senior FO:

You can possibly go a bit to the left. I agree that we're not in manual, eh?

The senior FO suggested changing course a little to the left to avoid turbulence they could see on their weather radar, and they altered the heading to a setting minus twelve degrees off their preset route.

–00:01:24 Junior FO:

What's that smell now?

–00:01:22 Senior FO:

It's... it's ozone.

–00:01:21 Junior FO:

It's ozone—that's it. We're all right.

–00:00:19

[Background noise increases]

Other A330-340 pilots identified it as typical noise of impact of ice crystals. Neither pilot alluded to it. The BEA noted that at the time pilots had little knowledge regarding the phenomenon. Nevertheless, Robert (the PNF) took it upon himself to reduce the airspeed down toward Mach 0.8 and switched on the engine anti-icing, no doubt in response to the indication of ice shown by the instruments.

–0:00:02 to 00:00

[Cavalry charge warning that autopilot is disengaging]

THE GLITCH (00:00:00) [02:10:05 UTC]

AUTOPILOT DISENGAGES AND BONIN TAKES OVER

00:00:01 Junior FO Bonin, the pilot flying (PF):

I have the controls.

00:00:03 Senior FO Robert, the pilot not flying (PNF):

All right.

Unlike Boeing airliners, which have traditional control columns that move in unison on both sides of the cockpit, Airbuses have sidesticks with no mechanical or simulated interconnection. In addition, as these are located on the coming on the far side of the pilots, it is very difficult for the other pilot to see what his colleague is doing, and particularly so in relative darkness.

Apparently, Robert had his seat set right back making it even more difficult to see what Bonin was doing with his stick.

Thus, the senior FO did not see that the PF had pulled back his stick and put the aircraft into a rapid climb. Without application of more power, the aircraft could only achieve this climb by using up kinetic energy in the form of airspeed and soon lost so much that it was in danger of stalling.

00:00:05 Two SV (synthetic voice) stall warnings (BEA calls it Stall 1 warning)

> *Stall.*
> *Stall.*

00:00:06 Senior FO:

> *What is that?*

Even so, the junior FO was still for some reason keeping the nose up, thus preventing the aircraft from diving and regaining essential airspeed.

00:00:08 Two SV stall warnings, last one truncated

> *Stall, s—*

00:00:09 Junior FO:

> *We haven't got a good display . . .*

00:00:10 Junior FO:

> *We haven't got a good display . . . . . . of speed.*

00:00:11 Senior FO:

> *We've lost the speeds . . .*

00:00:17 Senior FO:

> *Alternate law, protections law/Low/Lo.*

The CVR transcriber could not tell what Robert had said, so it is most unlikely Bonin had. In fact, what the ECAM had spelt out was "LOST." Over such a *crucial point* Robert should have insisted on confirmation that Bonin understood protections had been lost.

Worse, while Robert was speaking, Bonin was trying to make a point about the thrust levers. An example of bad CRM, having the two of them talking at the same time.

00:00:19 to 00:00:23 Senior FO:

Wait, we're losing . . .Wing anti-ice. Watch your speed. Watch your speed.

00:00:23 Junior FO:

Okay, Okay, Okay. I'm going back down.

00:00:26 Senior FO:

Go back down.

00:00:27 Senior FO:

According to that we're going up. According to all three you're going up, so go back down.

00:00:30 Junior FO:

Okay.

00:00:31 Senior FO:

You're at . . . Go back down.

00:00:37 Junior FO:

We're in a . . . We're in a climb.

00:00:45 Senior FO:

* * *, *where is he?*

It seems the senior FO had already called the captain. Anyway, from this time onward, he tried several times to call him back, and this must have drawn his attention away from what the junior FO was doing at this most critical time.

00:00:46

[Almost-continuous stall warnings start] (BEA calls them Stall 2 warnings)

00:01:01 Senior FO:

* * *, where is he?

Bonin (the PF) made slight nose-down inputs alternately to the right and to the left. The rate of climb, which was astounding for that great height with thin air had reached seven thousand feet a minute, had dropped to seven hundred feet a minute, and the roll varied between twelve degrees to the right and ten degrees to the left. The airspeed shown on the left side increased suddenly to 215 knots (Mach 0.68), while the speed displayed on the left primary flight display (PFD) remained invalid for twenty-nine seconds.

By then the aircraft was at an altitude of about 37,500 feet and the recorded angle of attack around four degrees. Stall 2 warnings continue.

00:01:05 Aircraft ultimately reaches a maximum height of 37,924 feet

00:01:20 Senior FO:

Do you understand what's happening or not?

00:01:28 Junior FO:

I don't have control of the airplane anymore now.

00:01:30 Junior FO:

I don't have control of the airplane at all.
Repetitive Stall 2 warnings continue.

00:01:37 Return of the Captain

[Noise of cockpit door opening.]
The captain's return to the cockpit coincided with the aircraft mushing downwards through 35,000 feet, the altitude it had been when he had departed a little earlier. Apart from the alarms and the senior FO's expression of concern, a quick glance at the altimeter might have led him to believe that not much had changed. He was not to know that the A330 had climbed almost 3,000 feet without added power and could really be stalling.

Captain:

Er, what are you [doing]?

00:01:39 Senior FO:

What's happening? I don't know, I don't know what's happening.

00:01:42 Junior FO:

We're losing control of the aircraft there.

00:01:39 Senior FO:

We lost all control of the aircraft. We don't understand anything. We've tried everything.

00:01:48 Captain:

So take that.

00:01:50 Senior FO:

Take that, take that.

00:01:53 Junior FO:

I have a problem; it's that I don't have vertical speed indication.

In fact, the aircraft was dropping so fast the indicator could not show the actual sink rate, though there was a colored mark indicating it was "off the dial."

00:01:59 Junior FO:

I have the impression that we have some crazy speed, no? What do you think?

The cacophony generated by the aircraft mushing downwards, with the air howling as it splayed off the wings, may have given the FO the impression they were traveling too fast, and needed the air brakes.

00:01:42 Senior FO:

No, above all don't extend [the air brakes].

00:02:09 Senior FO:

What do you think about it? What do you think? What do we need to do?

00:02:10 Captain:

I don't know, it's going down. [Impossible to translate colloquial "there" that the captain added, and the junior FO starts using too. Some exchanges omitted.]

00:02:22 Senior FO (with stall alarm still sounding):

You're climbing.

00:02:23 Senior FO (stall alarm still sounding):

You're going down, down, down.

Captain:

   * * * [Going down]

00:02:25 Junior FO:

   Am I going down now?

00:02:27 Senior FO:

   Go down.

Captain:

   No, you climb there.

00:02:34 Junior FO:

   Okay, we're in TOGA.

TOGA (takeoff/go-around) is a button that sets the engines to high power, and the control surface configuration, so that when in dense air at low altitude the aircraft can immediately climb out and away. It can also stop the aircraft stalling. However, at high altitude where the air is thin, the situation is quite different. Maximum thrust has hardly any effect, and with plenty of height to play with, the first requirement is to get the nose down so the aircraft dives and gains airspeed.

00:02:37 Junior FO:

   On alti what do we have here?

00:02:39 Stall warnings ongoing.
Captain:

   ***, it's impossible.

The junior FO again asked about altitude, without getting a reply, and in the following twenty seconds the captain's main concern was to tell him to get the wings horizontal, as the synthetic voice stall warnings continued.

00:03:13 Junior FO:

We're there, we're there, we're passing level one hundred [ten thousand feet].

00:03:20 Junior FO:

What is . . .? How come we're continuing to go right down now?

The stall warnings ceased when the airspeed fell below sixty knots because the creators of the software wanted to avoid it giving spurious stall warnings when landing and taking off. They could never imagine pilots would ever allow airspeed to fall so low in normal flight.

The odd result in this context was that when the pilots did something right, such as raising the airspeed above sixty knots, the warnings would restart, possibly making them think their action might be wrong. (Even when the airspeed was somewhat above sixty knots, the angle of attack meant the airspeed registered by the sensors would be less.)

00:03:35 Junior FO:

But I've been in maxi nose-up for a while.

This remark makes the captain *finally* realize what the junior FO has been doing wrong all along.

00:03:38 Captain:

No, no, no, don't climb.

00:03:40 Senior FO:

So, give me the controls; the controls to me; the controls to me.

00:03:41 Junior FO:

Go ahead. You have the controls. We are still in TOGA, eh.

00:03:50

With the senior FO taking control, the stall warnings recommenced even though the situation was improving, as explained above. With them dropping at around ten thousand feet per minute and little height remaining, it was too late anyway.

00:04:00 Captain:

Watch out, you're pitching up there.

00:04:02 Junior FO:

Well, we need to; we are at four thousand feet.

00:04:11 SV (synthetic voice) sink rate warning

[The "Pull up!" warning continues until the aircraft hits the sea.]

00:04:21 Impact with the Sea

The recordings stopped at two hours, fourteen minutes, and twenty-eight seconds UTC, that is *four minutes and twenty-one seconds* after the autopilot disconnect.

The last recorded values were:

Vertical speed: −10,912 feet a minute
Ground speed: 107 knots
Pitch attitude: 16.2 degrees nose-up
Roll angle: 5.3 degrees left
Magnetic heading: 270 degrees.

Though some of the passengers, not forgetting the cabin crew, would have been aware something was wrong, the fact that the nose was pointing upwards may have reassured them. The deceleration on hitting the sea, with the aircraft dropping at 10,912 feet a minute, would have been so great that they would have lost consciousness instantaneously.

THE NINE FACETS OF THE DISASTER

Facet 1: Junior First Officer Bonin (PF)

The BEA investigators tentatively attributed the abruptness of Bonin's stick input to the "startle effect" of suddenly having to take over and lack of experience/training for manual flying at that great height.

They also suggested he might have climbed because the icing-up of the pitot tubes had caused the altimeter to erroneously show a drop of a few hundred feet below its programmed thirty-five-thousand-foot cruising height, a deviation which would be indicated by an audible alert. Also, they said earlier repeated exchanges with the captain showed Bonin was fixated on the need to fly higher, and the sight of clear sky above might have reinforced this.

What little practice Bonin had of flying manually most likely involved following the flight director. Later, when the flight director bars reappeared, the investigators thought Bonin might out of habit blindly followed them, although with it simply reacting to changes in g and believing the steep climb and precipitous drop were intended, it was not telling them how to recover.

Perhaps the most plausible reason for Bonin's unbelievably steep climb, at least initially, and one highlighted by psychologists using sophisticated terms such as "cognitive tunneling," was that, not practiced in keeping the wings level under manual control in alternate law at high altitude, he became so mentally consumed by that delicate task that he simply did not realize he was climbing so steeply. Bear in mind that when the captain did eventually arrive, he too was primarily concerned with Bonin keeping the wings level and not the pitch.

As William Langewiesche so rightly points out in a piece for the October 2014 edition of *Vanity Fair*, the French pilots' unions take a very hard stand defending colleagues killed in the performance—or one might say—in the nonperformance of their duties. They say publishing what is on a cockpit voice recorder is an infringement of their deceased colleagues' human rights, though the pilots in question may well have brought about their own deaths and those of hundreds of passengers and crew.

Though ostensibly high-minded, the unions' thereby cow the French investigators into not revealing general poor conduct or incompetency. The BEA perhaps for that reason tell us little about Bonin, or the other two aircrew for that matter.

Some on the ***pprune.org*** website have said that as a former cabin attendant, like the captain, Bonin had not had to take the usual psychological tests prior to being taken on as a potential pilot.

Before going for his rest, the captain handed over authority to Bonin in a most perfunctory manner, even, unbelievably, having to confirm as an afterthought that the junior first officer was qualified (to make the landing in Paris, or perhaps take command).

Admittedly, the Air France protocol (since changed) for the handover was not well-thought-out and implied the pilot flying was also in charge, even though he might be the less experienced of the two.

The BEA said this resulted in the perverse situation where on one level Bonin deferred to Robert, without Robert having executive authority on another level. One commentator has even suggested that while Bonin was vocally acknowledging Robert's recommendations, his actions bore no relation to them—perhaps akin to someone being nagged by a spouse and saying "Yes, yes, dear," and doing whatever they want.

The BEA investigators did not pick up on Bonin not wanting to follow the captain's suggestion that he rest or catnap at his seat, since keeping awake all the way to Paris "would be hard on him." Robert, too, seemed concerned about Bonin's condition, which suggests there must have been some good reason for that. Could some other factor, say excess caffeine, with its five-hour half-life, found in some soft drinks in Brazil, have made him highly strung and twitchy?

One can never know.

Finally, Bonin alluded at the beginning and toward the end to them being in TOGA (takeoff go-around mode), evidently believing it would obviate a stall, which was not the case at high altitude. As said, Robert had also unforgivably not made clear to him normal protections were lost.

Facet 2: Senior First Officer Robert (PNF)

Robert was unable to assume command because Air France handover protocols at the time inferred the pilot flying (PF) was in charge. Also, he may have been undermined by the cozy relationship established between the captain and Bonin following the helicopter tour of Rio the two had taken with their women on the day of departure. Had he not only taken command, but also taken over the controls it is unlikely he would have made that disastrous climb. There would have been no stall, and as the aircraft moved into more clement conditions the ice in the pitot tubes would have melted and everything returned to normal.

Robert could see that the aircraft was climbing in the half minute following Bonin's assumption of manual control, telling him several times, without significant effect, to go down. Thirty-one seconds into the incident, seeing they were still climbing, he reiterated his wish that Bonin go down, but instead of making sure Bonin did so, he diverted his attention to calling the captain.

Showing his frustration at the captain's tardiness, Robert exclaimed, "Where the heck is he?" at +00:46 and +01:01 against the background of the repetitive stall warnings, to which he otherwise might have paid more attention.

This was the critical moment, wasted, when the situation was about to radically worsen. Maybe he felt only the captain could handle Bonin.

Four seconds later the aircraft reached its apogee, and having run out of kinetic energy, its airspeed decayed. Hanging there, it began to truly stall despite a couple of desultory nose-down inputs from Bonin.

The lack of airspeed also meant the A330 did not easily respond to stick inputs, so when Robert asked Bonin at +01:20, one minute twenty seconds after the autopilot disengagement, whether he knew what was happening, Bonin answered he no longer had control of the aircraft, repeating himself ten seconds later.

How could Robert, after an almost 3,000-foot climb in thin air, not have even given some credence to the stall warnings we shall never know. Furthermore, he had his seat set far back, as if he were just a casual observer, and his seat, later found in that position, stayed back. It made it more difficult for him to see what Bonin was doing. Was it so the captain could more easily take his place?

Though Robert, as a graduate of the ENAC (National School of Civil Aviation), was considered part of the elite and assumed to be supremely qualified by commentators, his course at the institution had been in the field of air traffic control. In consequence, though an experienced pilot, he had no special knowledge concerning the operation of computer-controlled aircraft. Prior to the trip to Rio, he had not even landed an A330 for almost three months, and with piloting not being his role at Air France, he might not have been assiduously trying to learn everything possible in that domain.

There is something to be said for the "captain" not taking over and concentrating on the thinking, but in this case, Robert who was meant to be doing the thinking and analysis was not only distracted from that by repeatedly calling the captain, but any deduction was negated by Bonin not following his advice, or worse, making him believe he was doing so when doing the opposite.

Facet 3: Captain Dubois

By deciding early in the flight not to alter course to avoid the storms, the captain in a sense set up the scenario that produced the glitch. Admittedly, it was allegedly Air France policy not to load significant extra fuel for major diversions to avoid storms on those Rio flights.

According to a mutual woman friend of both the captain and his veteran flight attendant-opera singer companion, who was to have joined them on the jaunt to Rio but missed the outbound flight because of indisposition, he was greatly looking forward to the three-day shared layover as a release from the stress at home related to his divorce. One can surmise that on the return flight, in addition to being extremely tired the captain would have been euphoric and perhaps more likely than usual to "not let some cumulonimbus mess them around." Other aircraft that night had changed course to avoid such storms.

According to a medical expert, his lack of sleep would have put him at times in a soporific state, with his faculties diminished like a drunk, especially on returning to the cockpit after relaxing and going into a quasi-sleep. Bill Palmer, author of *Understanding Air France 447*, thinks the captain was not in the rest station and returned to the cockpit because of the strange behavior of the aircraft, for instead of asking what was happening, he had said, "Err, what are you [doing]?"

If true—the discreet French investigators did not belabor this point—this means his return was delayed because he was most likely with his companion. Admittedly, any pilot might go back to chat with the flight attendants in the galley before taking his or her rest. Nonetheless, it was perhaps one of many factors contributing to the disaster, in that when he did finally return to the cockpit, the aircraft was mushing downward through the altitude it had been when he departed.

For a moment, he might have thought nothing much had really happened in the interim. Had he returned some thirty seconds earlier, the aircraft would have been at its apogee, making him perhaps realize what was happening and that the stall warnings were continuously sounding for good reason. Even fifteen seconds earlier could have made a significant difference.

Only at the very end, when Bonin told him he had been in "maxi nose-up for a while," did the captain realize—too late—what had been happening and tell him not to climb. Considering the captain's sleep deficit, even that was quite a feat.

To be fair to him, it would be difficult for anyone to properly assess the situation without having been told they had just made what was at that altitude a ridiculously steep climb. But, even if he had, was he in good enough shape with his lack of sleep to take over aggressively and appropriately?

A retired British Airways captain who used to fly that route from Rio de Janeiro has said he would never have gone for his rest before entering the potentially dangerous intertropical convergence zone, something that was accepted practice for Air France captains.

Had the captain been in his bunk next to the cockpit and returned sooner, Robert would not have diverted his attention for so long away from monitoring the aircraft and perhaps would have made sure Bonin was complying with his advice.

Facet 4: CRM—Culture of the Airline

After the overrun of an Air France A340 at Montreal in 2005, the freelance French aviation writer François Hénin said the airline was making serious efforts to rectify the easygoing attitude of its aircrew.

William Langewiesche, in the perceptive *Vanity Fair* article mentioned above, inferred that at Air France the egalitarian discipline of CRM had devolved into a self-indulgent style of flying. Though verbally confirming actions with one's colleague may seem unnecessary in normal circumstances, getting into the habit of doing so means one is much more likely to do so in a crisis. Some pilots at Air France may have been somewhat lax in this regard and lost the habit.

Although "cognitive tunneling"—too concerned with keeping the wings level to consider anything else—may at the outset have been the key factor, Bonin should later have made it clear to Robert he was pulling back on his stick, and, as said, only mentioned that to the captain right at the end, indicating he was aware of what he had been doing.

As said, Robert did not even confirm Bonin understood they had lost the usual protections such as stall protection, and in fact did not finish his phrase.

Adding to the confusion was the fact that once the aircraft lost airspeed and ceased responding immediately to sidestick inputs, statements or interrogative remarks by Robert, such as "You are going up/down," did not correlate with movements of Bonin's sidestick. For Bonin to push the nose down, he would have had to push his sidestick forward and maintain it there for some time, perhaps reducing engine thrust to stop it levering the nose up.

Facet 5: Stall Warnings Not Heeded

The crash occurred because the aircraft stalled, but at no point did any of the pilots mention the word "stall," though at one stage Robert said, "What's that?" when the warning sounded without making clear to what he was referring. These stall warnings went on for a very long time, and the captain must have heard them even though they stopped soon after his arrival when the airspeed fell below sixty knots, as explained.

The BEA and others point out that when a stall warning sounds in normal flying conditions, it is usually of little concern to the pilots, as the computer—under normal law—is always there to protect them. Also, it is very possible Bonin thought the stall situation was covered, as he twice says, as if reassuring himself, that they are in the TOGA (takeoff/go-around) configuration, which at low altitude (but not high) would normally get them out of a stall.

As mentioned elsewhere, it has been suggested that sounds tend to get mentally filtered out in crises. However, the stall warnings did sound seventy-five times in all so could hardly have passed unnoticed.

Facet 6: Pilot-Machine Interface

The BEA report euphemistically refers to the pilot-machine interface as ergonomics, when in fact they give it a much broader meaning.

For anyone particularly interested in the pilot-machine interface facet of this incident, we must again recommend *Understanding Air France 447*, by Bill Palmer.

Particularly interesting is the way Palmer explains the great gulf between flying an Airbus A330 in normal and alternate law.

Sullenberger and others, and the BEA, have mentioned possible improvements, not all really coming under ergonomics:

1. There should be a clear indication of the reason that the autopilot disengages of its own accord. This should be shown on the ECAM, as should stall warnings—in addition to the audible ones. This would have meant the pilots would not only have faced less uncertainty but, perhaps more

importantly, would have meant the pilot not flying (PNF) could have concentrated on what the aircraft was doing rather than wasting time trying to fathom what was happening and reading out irrelevant messages appearing on the ECAM.

2. In a crisis, humans pay more attention to visual cues than to aural cues, which are often lost among a cacophony of other aural warnings, and there should be a visual cue in addition to the one on the airspeed indicator tape, which was not valid anyway.

3. Following on from the previous point, airliners should be equipped with an instrument showing the angle of attack, which would confirm the stall and give pilots a better indication of what is happening. Its installation on certain military aircraft apparently significantly reduced accidents. However, getting the angle of attack indicator to provide useful information it not simple as stalling speed depends very much on height.

4. As already mentioned, the sidesticks do not move in unison, making it difficult if not impossible for the PNF to see what the PF is doing, and notably something silly. Some means of indicating this should not be difficult. Likewise, the throttles do not move to remind pilots of what the engines have been told to do. Eliminating such features has some pluses, but the case needs to be argued. Interestingly, though Boeing are resolutely sticking to their control column concept, more users,

military, high-end business jet users, and now civil, are favoring the sidestick, and notably "active Sidesticks." These not only enable the pilot flying to better feel what he is doing, but also allow the other pilot to see or feel what he or she is doing and might well have enabled Robert to prevent Bonin making that disastrous climb in the first place.

Airbus ironically may be right in that, after proper training, the pilot-machine improvements proposed, though in theory desirable, may not be needed to prevent an absurd repeat.

Facet 7: Air France Training

The BEA very much exculpates the pilots because Air France had not trained them to cope with such a situation at high altitude. Post disaster, Air France, not to mention many other airlines, have been training their pilots to handle high-altitude upsets and stalls and how to avoid them in the first place.

Facet 8: Pitot Probes and Choice Thereof

The icing-up of the pitot tubes supplied by the French conglomerate Thales—intent on ousting the US makers of such equipment who had gained a stranglehold after World War 2—also provided the trigger for the disaster, and Air France should have replaced them, and were in the process of doing so.

However, the disaster resulted from the way the two first officers mishandled the situation. Other instances where the pitot tubes had iced up had been handled competently, though in many of those cases it was daylight and the pilots had more visual references.

Anyway, in the year or so prior to the disaster we are discussing, Air France had nine instances of problems with the A330 and A340 pitot probes and was changing them.

Facet 9: Investigative and Supervisory Bodies—BEA, DGAC, and EASA

When the BEA announced that while the pitot tubes may well have been a factor in the crash, but were surely not the only factor, the Air France pilots' union said it was only trying to cover up its own failures and those of the DGAC (French Directorate General of Civil Aviation). The argument was that it had failed to pick up on problems with the Thales pitot tubes, and the European Air Safety Agency had not been diligent in applying the latest lessons in certifying them.

The BEA report said the A330s had originally been fitted with Goodrich probes, but the DGAC, on finding some problems, ordered that they be fitted with a more advanced Goodrich probe or with the Thales probe that iced up on AF447. Thus, the French DGAC opened the door for the Thales probe, but Air France was still responsible for going through with it, perhaps with Thales being very persuasive.

Private Matters
and the Relationship Between First Officers

Because we think they had a material bearing on the disaster, we have alluded to private matters one would not normally divulge.

Firstly, the ones leading to the captain's sleep deficit, and even his very likely euphoric and soporific frame of mind when early in the flight he just might have bothered to adjust course to avoid the storms, as did the captains of other airliners that night.

Bill Palmer's fascinating book, *Understanding Air France 447*, dismissed our point regarding the captain's supposed fatigue as unproven and high-mindedly focused on the technical aspects, all the while suggesting fatigue on the part of the two first officers may have been a factor, which of course could be even more pertinent.

However, Bill Palmer was possibly not aware at the time of writing that the French investigators had not revealed that the captain *himself* had said on the CVR that he had only had an hour's sleep and it was not enough. One can understand them expunging him pronouncing they were going to die, but apparently the language overall on the CVR was more vulgar and ultimately panic-stricken than the BEA made public. But surely the mention of lack of sleep cannot be regarded as a private matter.

Secondly, for what it's worth, an aviation expert familiar with Air France culture and much else told the author that Robert and Bonin hated each other, and that this is even evident from nuances in the "sanitized" version of the CVR. When talking to the captain, Bonin referred to Robert (who was having his rest) as "he" rather than using his first name, at the very least suggesting he was an outsider.

The awkward atmosphere could have prevented Robert relaxing properly during that rest and led Bonin to spurn his advice and even do the opposite. Robert was from the academic elite and part of management, in contrast to Bonin, whose engagement as a pilot had been via a much humbler route.

While the captain's questionable comportment underlay the disaster, it was the two first officers at the coalface who turned what was a mere glitch into a disaster. Their relationship is therefore very relevant.

Interestingly, Bill Palmer makes the point that yaw damping, still functioning in alternate law, probably prevented the aircraft flipping over under Bonin's control.

Unlikely to Recur

Lessons learnt should mean that never again will there be such a stall following a high-altitude autopilot disengagement due a loss of credible airspeed data. Pilots will be reminded that all they need do—apart from keeping the wings level (not easy without the computer) and continuing to fly level at the already proven power setting—is *nothing*.

They are also being taught how to recover from a high-altitude stall should one ever occur.

The Future—Artificial Intelligence (AI)

Research is being done on an autopilot featuring artificial intelligence that can, for instance, guesstimate airspeed from more data sources, such as GPS and inertial guidance systems, before "giving up" and disengaging. The team developing it found it could even learn from experience gained on different models of aircraft. That would apply to cases where pilots had flown on manually with no problems after the autopilot disengaged due to lack of airspeed data.

Such an autopilot could continue, as the lawyers say, "under advisement" and avoid the pilots being thrown in at the deep end, where the startle effect and lack of manual flying dexterity are liable to make them do more harm than good, as tragically happened here.

The Causes Were Complex

AF447 is frequently cited as a prime example of a crash due to automation making pilots lose their flying skills.

While Bonin had not demonstrated good flying skills, the crash was also the product of many other unfortunate human and technical factors.

To start with, on that night, other captains were not so dismissive about storms and routed their aircraft to avoid them.

It need never have happened.

By "Pull Down!" Captain Did Not Mean Pull Stick (Java Sea, 2014)

Confusion over language perhaps sealed their fate

> An intermittent fault of no great consequence had meant pilots had to repeatedly reset a system. On the fourth time that flight, the captain tried a novel technique, not realizing the consequences of switching off the computer.
>
> AirAsia Flight 8501, December 28, 2014

The A320 on the AirAsia two-hour flight from Juanda International Airport, Surabaya, Indonesia to Singapore had 166 people, 155 passengers and 7 crew on board when it took off virtually on schedule at 5:35 in the morning.

The captain was fifty-three-year-old Iriyanto, a former Indonesian Air Force officer with a total of 20,537 flying hours, 6,100 of which were with Indonesia AirAsia on the Airbus A320. The copilot was forty-six-year-old First Officer Rémi Emmanuel Plesel, a French national born in Martinique. He had a total of 2,247 flying hours with Indonesia AirAsia.

The aircraft seemed to be in good order, except that for almost a year the rudder travel limit unit (RTLU) had an intermittent fault that had manifested itself twenty-seven times, both in the air and on the ground. The RTLU is a unit that prevents the rudder being moved too far in flight and perhaps breaking off, as happened at Queens, New York, when the pilot made excessive rudder movement while caught up in wake turbulence.

Instead of repairing the RTLU fault properly—it was due to a badly soldered connection in a circuit board—

the system had simply been reset, at least twenty-three times in all. Just three days earlier, the captain had seen how, when it failed on the ground, the mechanic first rebooted it, and when that did not work, he tripped and reset the circuit breakers for the main computer. When the captain asked the maintenance personnel whether it would be okay to do that in-flight if the problem came back, they assured him it would.

While this was okay on the ground, it was not in-flight, as it would lead to a series of computers being disabled, including those for autopilot and autothrottle, with the aircraft passing into alternate law without most of the safety protections.

At 6:12, with the aircraft flying at their allotted cruise altitude of thirty-two thousand feet over the Java Sea, the pilots saw a storm ahead and requested permission to climb to thirty-eight thousand feet. This request was denied because of other aircraft in the vicinity, although they were allowed to alter course to the left.

An alarm then sounded indicating failure of the RTLU. The first officer being the pilot flying told the captain to see what ECAM action should be taken. The ECAM (electronic centralized aircraft monitor) is a monitor (screen) like a super-checklist that tells the pilots what to do in various situations, prioritizing problems according to urgency.

In this case, it told the pilots to reboot two of the flight augmentation computers (FACs). The warning disappeared after the captain had done that.

A minute or so later, the same thing happened, and the captain again followed the identical ECAM instructions, with the warning disappearing. They contacted air traffic control at 6:14 and were given authorization to climb to thirty-four thousand feet, which they did not acknowledge, perhaps because the alarm had gone off again, requiring the captain to go through the same sequence of actions. When they might have been about to confirm their climb authorization, the alarm went off a fourth time. Exasperated, the captain said, "Enough with this."

Though the first officer said, "Follow the ECAM," as before, the captain said he had a better idea and tripped the two circuit breakers. This stopped the warning, just as it had done on the ground, but not only that: the autopilot disengaged, and the aircraft passed into alternate law, meaning the normal law protections such as those preventing stalling even under manual control were lost. The A320 rolled to the left.

The captain, who had been standing in order to operate the circuit breakers, returned to his seat and in doing so noticed the aircraft rolling, and said, "Level, level, level."

The first officer, having inexplicably allowed the roll to continue for nine seconds without intervening, turned to the right, and overbanked to the right. He then overbanked to the left, putting the aircraft into a steep climb of six thousand feet per minute—twice what would be normal.

This seemed to be similar to what Bonin did in AF447, in that so preoccupied was he with managing the lateral stability that he inadvertently climbed more than he should have.

Captain:

Pull down, pull down, pull down!

The first officer evidently thought he meant he should pull back on his sidestick, though the captain must have meant pull the nose down—one does not really pull a sidestick *down*. The aircraft climbed five thousand feet in fifty-four seconds to an altitude of thirty-seven thousand feet, the opposite of what the captain intended, for the flight data recorder later showed the captain had pushed his sidestick forward but forgotten to push his priority button, with the result that their inputs had canceled each other out and the aircraft continued to climb.

The aircraft finally stalled at that 37,000-foot apogee, banked deeply to the left, and dropped.

The captain again said, "Pull!"

Whatever that meant, pulling on the sidesticks perhaps was not the way to recover.

The captain could have had full control himself and not concerned himself with the first officer simply by pressing the red priority button on his sidestick. Though it has been said the priority button has to be held down for forty seconds, that is only to latch it, meaning it no longer needs to be pressed to maintain priority. Incidentally, the priority button can also be used to take control from the autopilot.

The Search

Disappearing from Jakarta radar at twenty-four thousand feet, the A320 plunged into the Java Sea, with no possibility of survivors, though of course controllers could not be sure of that at the time.

A massive search was undertaken using aircraft and ships from many nations. Fishermen had seen some wreckage, but it was only on returning to shore the next morning that they were able to tell the authorities where to look. Search aircraft sighted wreckage on December 30 very close to where the Jakarta radar had shown they had come down.

Over the following days, wreckage and bodies were retrieved from the surface, and on January 3 wreckage was found on the seafloor. Within ten days the flight data recorder and cockpit voice recorder had both been recovered.

Because of the bad weather at the time of the crash, and the controllers' refusal to allow the A320 to climb over it due to congestion, everyone was assuming stormy weather was the cause, with even the sudden climb attributed to an incredible updraft—in the intertropical convergence zone, renowned for fickle weather. The recorders were able to show that was not the case and that the accident happened as described above.

The Investigation

As it was not a US-built aircraft, the NTSB, who had disagreed with the Indonesians over the SilkAir 737 crash, were not part of the investigation, which was led by Indonesia's National Transportation Safety

Committee (NTSC), with the assistance of Australia, France, Malaysia, and Singapore.

Although Singapore had granted AirAsia the right to fly that route daily, the Indonesians had only granted rights for fewer days and not for Sundays. The flight had, from their point of view, been operating illegally.

The flight data recorder had shown the weather was not the cause. Regarding the actions of the crew, the investigators were surprised that following the disengagement of the autopilot it took nine seconds for the first officer, who was the pilot flying, to correct the yaw and bank caused by the rudder being no longer under control by the computer. Letting the situation get so extreme, a bank angle of fifty-four degrees, might have contributed to his sense of panic and led him to overcompensate and forget he was climbing excessively.

The crux was miscommunication between the two pilots caused by the captain saying, "Pull down" when he must have meant pull the nose down, not pull the sidestick back. The report recommended that work should be done on establishing standard terminology for such things.

Had the computer not been disabled, it would have prevented the copilot doing the wrong thing.

Chapter 18
SINGULAR CASES

Plane Fell from the Sky, with Pilots' Reputation (Saginaw, 1979)

A murky affair where it seems pilot treated unfairly

> Because it was only an "incident," with no loss of life, and the aircraft was immediately repaired, thus destroying the evidence, it was not investigated as rigorously as it might have been.
>
> TWA Flight 841, April 4, 1979

The fourteen-year-old TWA Boeing 727 trijet took off from New York's JFK airport at 8:25 p.m. bound for Minneapolis–Saint Paul with eighty-two passengers and seven crew. They did not have far to go, but a very strong headwind meant it would take longer than usual. To save fuel and have a smoother flight, the pilots decided to climb from thirty-five thousand to thirty-nine thousand feet, though flying at that great height was more delicate.

They and the passengers found the flight much smoother; moreover, the headwind had fallen from above one hundred to eighty-five knots.

There were three people in the cockpit. Forty-four-year-old Captain Harvey Gibson was nicknamed "Hoot" because he had once played the part of an owl in a school play, which involved running across the stage shouting, "Hoot! Hoot! Hoot!"[1]

Before joining TWA, he had been in the Marine Corps for two years to support a young wife and children, been an air traffic controller at Chicago Midway Airport, and had spent a year as a pilot at a company flying Hugh Hefner and Playboy bunnies around the US.

He was qualified to fly not only the Boeing 727 but also the DC-9, Lockheed 1011 Tristar, and the Boeing 747, having in fact been flying the jumbo as first officer for the experience and to enjoy flying the long-haul, and more exciting, routes. He had been off work for three months due to a broken ankle and had just returned as a 727 captain after three weeks of ground training and route checks. He had allegedly told his two colleagues to keep an eye on him, as it was his first time back on the 727 as captain, which would suggest it would be most unlikely he would risk doing anything unconventional, especially at very high altitude, where margins between going too fast and too slow are slim.

His copilot was First Officer Kennedy, who had served for eight years as a flight engineer on joining TWA eleven years earlier, before becoming a first officer pilot. He had a total of 10,336 flying hours, of which 8,348 had been on the 727, and was no novice.

The flight engineer, which any sizable airliner had to have in those days, was thirty-seven-year-old Second Officer Banks, who, though a qualified commercial pilot, had worked as a flight engineer for nine years. He had also served in the military.

The Upset According to the Pilots

With the autopilot set to hold as they cruised at thirty-nine thousand feet, Hoot was rummaging in his flight bag for the charts for their next stop when there was a vibrating sensation in the rudder pedals, followed by buffeting that could be felt through the airframe. The instruments showed the aircraft was still flying with the wings level, but the autopilot had moved the control wheel twenty to thirty degrees to the left. This had not been noticed by his two colleagues, who were busy.

Taking over manual control, Hoot found he, too, had to maintain the control wheel over to the left. The aircraft then suddenly yawed to the right, then even more, until it developed into a roll and then a pitch downward, which Hoot tried to correct by applying full left aileron and pulling back on his stick, but to no apparent effect.

Application of full left rudder slowed the roll momentarily, but then, as the aircraft banked forty-five to sixty degrees to the right and seemed about to turn over, Hoot pulled the thrust levers back again, to no avail. The aircraft then turned over and pitched downward.

It plunged on and on down, and it seemed they were doomed. As a last resort, Hoot got his copilot to deploy the landing gear, even though that meant the gear doors would be ripped off in the slipstream. Whether it was because of the landing gear drag slowing the aircraft, or the rupture of hydraulic lines controlling a misbehaving rudder, or the greater controllability in thicker air, or a combination of all three, Hoot was finally able to pull the aircraft out of its dive, with it at moments having had to withstand 5 g without the wings breaking off.

How close to the ground the aircraft came is difficult to say. Officially, it was five thousand feet. Unofficially, it was much closer, even hundreds of feet—after landing Hoot found a tree branch in the undercarriage, but that might have been picked up afterward.

The pilots had not only survived a precipitous dive but had to bring the damaged aircraft back to an airport and land safely. The one they chose was a compromise. The nearest, Saginaw, only had short runways and limited facilities, and the favorite, Chicago, was too far away to risk going for in an aircraft that might become unflyable. They therefore opted for nearer Detroit, despite the weather not being so good there.

They did a low-level flyby, with rescue personnel shining searchlights on the landing gear, and were told by the tower that both were down, but the one on the right looked misaligned. Hoot came in fast at 205 knots and touched down perfectly on the left undercarriage, keeping the right one off the ground as long as possible. It held until they came to a stop but collapsed when a tractor began pulling the aircraft away from the runway, showing how close a shave it had been.

On being told fuel was leaking from the wings and that passengers should evacuate, the pilots decided to have them leave via the easily deployable stairs at the rear— an almost unique feature of the 727—without risking injury on the slides.

Only eight people on board were injured during the upset, partly because Hoot, knowing passengers would not have their seat belts fastened, had pulled back on his control column to maintain some positive g. In fact, when calm was restored a passenger gulped down the cocktail he had ordered, indicating that although the passengers had endured a terrifying experience, it was more like a roller coaster ride, and only the pilots knew how close to death they had been.

A passenger looked into the cockpit to thank the aircrew before exiting and noticed two of them staring ahead as if they were in shock, which might explain why they did not remember whether they had erased the cockpit voice recording (CVR). They were initially seen as heroes.

No Crash Site—Hence No Proper Investigation

Because there was no crash site and no need for deployment of the always on standby" go-team" consisting of NTSB staff with appropriate qualifications for specific roles, the incident was not properly investigated at the outset.

[This case of not having a proper investigation at the outset reminds one of a recent event that could have been truly calamitous, where the left runway at San Francisco was out of use and an Air Canada airliner in the dark almost touched down on the taxiway adjacent to the operating runway. On seeing the Air Canada aircraft unbelievably coming down the pilot of one of the five aircraft on the taxiway flashed his lights and the Air Canada airliner aborted the landing.

As there was no crash the incident was only investigated later by which time the cockpit voice recording showing the state of affairs in the Air Canada cockpit had been overwritten.]

In Hoot's case, officials working for the FAA and the NTSB then surreptitiously revealed to journalists that the CVR had been erased. Since the recorder ran on a half-hour loop to protect pilot privacy, and longer than that had been taken to get back to an airport and park, the CVR would not have included the upset or any of the time leading up to it. However, there remained the possibility they erased it to delete discussion of a cover-up, even though there would hardly have been time for that when bringing back a crippled aircraft with doubts as to whether the undercarriage would hold up.

Nevertheless, the press felt they were onto a good story.

Whether it was increasing pressure from the press, or out of a desire to stop pilots routinely erasing the CVRs, or a combination of both, the chairman of the NTSB took responsibility for the investigation away from their local technical man and put in charge an investigator whose qualifications were principally legal, ordering him to hold the initial formal deposition by the pilots in the presence of the press, something unheard of, as the media would normally only be present at the end of an investigation prior to issuance of the final report.

On the day of the deposition, a week after the incident, Hoot, copilot Kennedy, and First Officer Banks were not in good condition, having suffered from lack of sleep, the trauma of the near-death experience, and many difficult interviews.

Though the crew explained to those attending—NTSB and FAA staff, representatives from the pilots' union, TWA, and Boeing—what had happened, the focus switched to the question of the deletion of the DVR, with Hoot saying that he could not remember having done so, though he usually did. This led to the man from the FAA whose usual role was pursuing pilots for not following regulations obsessing on a line of questioning about whether erasing the CVR was permissible.

As a result, instead of the press properly reporting what pilots had said about what had happened, they focused their stories on the erasure of the CVR and what it might imply.

The legally-minded head investigator then latched on to a rumor that to save fuel, pilots of the 727 were flying it with two degrees of flap, having prevented the slats deploying by disengaging their circuit breakers. This scenario was given legs by a passenger way back in coach saying she had seen the flight engineer come into the cabin and hand food trays from the cockpit to a steward just before the incident.

This led the investigators to conclude that in the engineer's absence, the pilots had deployed two degrees of flap, but on his return, he had unsuspectingly reset the circuit breakers. When the pilots then retracted the flaps to retract the slats, the misaligned number seven slat failed to come back in, with the result the upset occurred.

The following comment, posted by Hipexec on the **https://pprune.org** pilots' website in September 2016 seems to prove this was a red herring:

> "The amazing thing about the Boeing suggestion about pulling circuit breakers and extending two degrees of trailing-edge flaps in cruise was I never—I mean never—discussed, much less contemplated, it during any one of my ten thousand hours on the 727. We constantly discussed ways of saving fuel but never talked about extending flaps in cruise.
>
> Where Boeing ever dug that one up is beyond me. If Boeing knew such a procedure would save fuel, why didn't they design a procedure so we could use it? It sounds to me like a big, fat CYA red herring to distract any litigation away from Boeing."

No one who had used the technique was ever found, and in 1980, flight tests by Boeing showed that rather than reducing fuel consumption the supposedly widely used technique increased it! The reason the rumor spread as it did may have been that, as we have said elsewhere in this book, "hero pilots" or prima donnas are not always popular with colleagues or even flight attendants, with some pilots who have skillfully saved their aircraft and passengers even preferring not to be officially commended in the knowledge that others have suffered or had their careers torpedoed after their feat became publicized.

Thereafter, the investigation locked on to this "Boeing Scenario," excluded other possibilities, and, unbelievably, did not question the pilots again, perhaps in the belief they would be lying. They did not even do simple things like interview the cabin crew to check the facts regarding the supposed handing over of the food trays by the flight engineer just prior to the upset. Neither did they ask them about the vibration and the yaw to the right mentioned by the pilots.

Although it was claimed wiring to the CVR had been checked to show only the pilots could have erased it, this was untrue. The flight data recorder only recorded a few parameters onto aluminum foil. When it did not seem to confirm the Boeing scenario, interpretations were altered. The FDR was anyway far too primitive to properly record the motions of an aircraft rolling over and did not record the positions of the controls or airfoils.

The investigators became locked into the idea that the pilots were guilty—otherwise, the 727 might have to be grounded—and focused on evidence suggesting that. The final report, with one member of the board reticent, declared the pilots must have been at fault.

The chief investigator was later promoted to administrative posts in the NTSB but never again served as an investigator. His appeal against a later demotion was denied on the grounds that "his performance did not demonstrate the excellence required to meet the goals of the special executive service of civilian government."

Justice Delayed, Justice Denied

Emilio Corsetti III has probably written the definitive book on the incident. Called *Scapegoat: A Flight Crew's Journey from Heroes to Villains to Redemption*, it looks in the upset and the resetting of the CVR.

He says the pilots were vindicated in the end, but this was only morally, for the long fight for justice had taken its physical and mental toll and was never legally won.

He seems to prove that the NTSB, after being sidetracked by the erasure of the CVR, the loss of the number seven slat, and the Boeing scenario, failed to consider the most likely causes, such as yaw damper and rudder problems.

In that respect, the case has some parallels with the longest-running NTSB investigation ever, that of the quirk of the rudder of the Boeing 737, described in Chapter 6, where the NTSB did not jump to conclusions— quite the opposite.

---

[1]A review on Amazon in the US by someone offended by our account of the shooting down of an airliner by the USS *Vincennes* ridiculed us for inventing this reason for the nickname Hoot.

We didn't. It's in Corsetti's authoritative book *Scapegoat*.

Not All Pilots Can Conduct Air Tests (Off French Med Coast, 2008)
A mere formality turned to disaster

> This highlights the danger of pilots who are not test pilots carrying out tests without defining what constitutes a pass or fail, and the problems a pilot can face on taking over manual control from the computer.
>
> XL Airways Flight 888T, November 27, 2008

Faced with a refusal by the air traffic controller at Bordeaux on the French Atlantic coast to allow them to engage in test flights in general air traffic, the pilots of the Airbus A320 had cut short their "acceptance flight" and turned back to Perpignan Airport on the Mediterranean. In just under an hour—half the time intended—they had surreptitiously managed to fit all but one of the tests into their flight plan without air traffic control objecting.

The pilot flying (PF) was XL Airways 51-year old Captain Kaepell with 12,709 flying hours, of which 7,038 were on that type of aircraft. His copilot was 58 with 5,525 hours on type.

Based in Frankfurt, they would have been tired, having taken a taxi at 4:30 that morning to catch the flight to Montpellier, 80 miles by car from Perpignan Airport where the A320 had been sent for final maintenance and paintwork before XL Airways returned it to Air New Zealand at the end of its two-year lease. Sitting behind them was Air New Zealand's Captain Horrell.

At 15:43:37, on their descent towards Perpignan Airport, Captain Kaepell disengaged the autopilot, saying in somewhat broken English:

Down below the clouds so you want what?

Captain Horrell replied:

To go slower you mean?

Kaepell reduced the thrust to idle, all the while keeping the nose down to maintain airspeed in accordance with the Perpignan controller's instructions. Their altitude at that point was 4,080 feet and their airspeed 166 knots.

The two pilots were evidently treating this more as a demonstration than a test for they were also busy explaining to the Perpignan controller that they did not want to do a full-stop landing but a go-around and proceed to Frankfurt.

Little did they know the demonstration could never work for in hosing down the fuselage mechanics had failed to cover the angle of attack sensors on the side. This had allowed water to penetrate deep inside the mechanism, that had frozen when the aircraft reached 31,000 feet locking two of the three sensors for the rest of the flight.

Besides making it impossible for the stall protections in normal law to work, it also meant $V_{\alpha PROT}$ and $V_{\alpha MAX}$ on the primary flight display speed strip were underestimated. "α" is the abbreviation Airbus use for angle of attack and $V_{\alpha PROT}$ is the airspeed at which the stall protections should come into play.

With full flap set and gear down, the A320 descended through 3,100 feet. Kaepell allowed the nose to rise, and the airspeed fell to 136 knots, then to 107 knots. At 15:45:05 the stall warning triggered with the pitch +18.6 degrees and airspeed 99 knots and Kaepell's sidestick still held slightly back. Treating it as an approach to stall, Kaepell applied go-around thrust and pushed his stick forward, but due to the load factor, not enough for the elevators to go beyond the neutral position to the stops and remove the extreme nose-up trim which unfortunately the computer had just set to enable the aircraft to fly so slowly.

Kaepell overcorrected a roll to the left producing a stalling sideslip to the right that engendered discrepancies in the air data. Not able to make sense of the situation, the fly by wire system switched to direct law. The investigators believe the pilots missed the aural warning of that because it was masked by the stall warning. Neither pilot seemed to have noticed "USE MANUAL PITCH TRIM" that also appeared in amber on the primary flight display.

The elevators (operated via the sidestick) could not overcome the combined effect of the pitch trim set at its maximum nose-up and the go-around thrust of engines set low down under the wings also levering the nose up.

We do not have space to give details of subsequent pilot inputs and the resultant behavior of the aircraft, only that by 15:45:42, after rising enough for the stall warning to stop momentarily, the airspeed had fallen to 40 knots. Two seconds later the maximum values recorded were a pitch of +57 degrees (i.e. exceedingly nose up), and an altitude of 3,788 feet, at which point the aircraft lurched over and careered down into the sea. All on board, including three Air New Zealand engineers and a New Zealand Civil Aviation Authority official in the passenger cabin, were killed.

Only sixty-two seconds had elapsed between the time the stall warning first triggered and the moment the recordings stopped!

The Investigation

This crash was very troubling because a month earlier another Airbus, a Qantas A330, had behaved very bizarrely (see Chapter 17) off the coast of Australia, albeit with the pilot managing to recover. After first suspecting the Air Data Inertial Reference Units as the Qantas A330 investigators had done, the French investigators were able to show the cause was the freezing of the water in the mechanisms of the two angle of attack sensors on the left of the fuselage. A third sensor still working was ignored by the system on the "odd man out" principle.

The investigators thought it likely that Horrell by saying "alpha floor, we're in manual" likely thought that the alpha floor function had triggered, and "manual" signified the autopilot had disconnected. They also note that the aircraft's lack of reaction to the nose-down control input did not draw the pilots' attention to the position of the horizontal stabilizer and the loss of the auto-trim function.

The pilots did not understand what was happening but had little time in which to do so. Earlier, as the airspeed dropped, they had not noticed $V_{\alpha PROT}$ and $V_{\alpha MAX}$ on the primary flight display speed band were unusual and low.

Other Factors:

1. The test should have been carried out at 14,000 feet.

2. What was a pass? What was a fail? If instead of relying solely on the calculations of the aircraft's computer, the lowest airspeed for initiation of the stall protection $V_{\alpha PROT}$ had been determined independently and had been kept in mind, the test would have been aborted in time.

3. Neither airline deemed it necessary to roster check captains for the task, let alone properly trained test pilots who always take precautions and for instance would never do such a test at low altitude.

Captain SandL on ***https://pprune.org*** sums up the situation very aptly:

I know that the major leasing companies ask for a "2-hour demonstration flight" but they do not specify what is included. Part of the reason may be that not all airlines have crew who are able to conduct a full air test.

Valuable lessons for Airbus and others

The official BEA (French Aviation Investigation and Analysis Bureau) final report did not analyze the fly-by-wire reactions—no G-trace. Nor did it speculate on how the pilots might have recovered had the test been done at 14,000 feet in accordance with the original plan. Though the last recorded values at 15:46:06.8, namely a pitch of -14 degrees, a bank angle of 15 degrees to the right, and an airspeed of 263 knots (and altitude of 340 ft) suggest that with a little more height to play with they could have easily recovered, the elevators were surprisingly in the nose-down position even though Kaepell was pulling back on his stick to raise the nose! The report says this was probably because a load factor higher than the value commanded leads to a nose-down movement of the elevator and a rapid rise in pitch is offset by the flight control law.

Appendix 10 of the BEA report, however, looks at how the computer systems functioned in flight and what data they considered or dismissed. It is extremely complicated and may not be worth studying at length as programming will surely have since been modified in the light of the lessons learned.

Designers and programmers of fly-by-wire systems must envisage all possibilities, however improbable. Though this impromptu low-speed test proved fatal for those on board, it provided lessons for pilots, Airbus and others that may well have saved lives on revenue flights.

Boeing 737 MAX Crashes

Lion Air Flight 610—737 MAX Indonesia (October 2018)
Ethiopian Airlines Flight 302 (March 2019)

When Boeing produced the MAX version, the larger diameter fuel-efficient engines had to be placed further forward increasing the risk of a stall. Without telling the pilots Boeing incorporated software to push the nose powerfully down in such an event.

At the time of writing, the aircraft have been grounded world-wide. Further details will be in Part 3 (Glossary and Updates) published in September 2019.

Landing Without Monitoring Airspeed (San Francisco, 2013)
777 was flying too slowly to climb over airport seawall

> This incident highlights not only the absolute no-no of allowing airspeed to fall too low but also the problems an evacuation can pose.
>
> Asiana Airlines Flight 214, July 6, 2013

Pilots had been notified in advance that the instrument landing system (ILS) for San Francisco's 28L left runway would be out of service. Without the ILS, pilots use the runway's visual precision approach path indicator (PAPI) to help them keep to the five-degree glide slope.

PAPI is a simple but reliable system whereby four lights set beside the runway threshold appear to change color according to the angle of approach. If the pilots are too high, there are more white lights than red; if they are on the glide path, there is an equal number of each; and if they are too low, there are more red than white.

All four lights were white, indicating the Boeing 777 from Inchon, South Korea, was too high as it came over the sea from afar to land on that runway on recovered land, with a facing of boulders capped by a low seawall.

Without ILS, the Asiana Airlines pilots could not use the Autoland system to keep them on the glide path. They were nevertheless using the autopilot to make the aircraft do what they wanted in terms of airspeed and rate of descent, but not altitude.

About three nautical miles from the runway, with them still too high, the pilot flying for some reason changed the autopilot mode to "Flight Level-Change." This made the autopilot latch on to the 3,000 feet that had been programmed for an eventual go-around and initiate a climb, not at all what the pilot wanted. To counter this, the PF disconnected the autopilot and pulled the thrust levers back to idle, putting the autopilot, unusually, in "Hold" mode, meaning it no longer controlled airspeed via the autothrottles.

Airspeed No Longer Controlled by Autothrottle

With the engines idling, the aircraft's glide slope steepened, and about 1.4 nautical miles from the runway they found themselves finally on the glide path and by chance virtually at the 137-knot target speed they had selected for the actual landing. Unknown to the pilots, the autothrottle was not responsible for that, as it was in "Hold" mode.

Apart from that perhaps easy misunderstanding, their sink rate was about 1,200 feet per minute, when it should have been 700.

The observer pilot had a few seconds earlier politely mentioned the sink rate but did not repeat the warning when, with them so near the ground, it was even more pertinent. One can only assume that all three pilots were so fixated on the PAPI lights turning to red that no one noticed the falling airspeed, though of course the pilot flying was pulling back on his control column, desperate to climb and get some white lights, but with less and less effect due to the falling airspeed.

Eleven seconds before reaching the seawall, there was an audible warning that their airspeed was too low. Four seconds later, with the airspeed at about 108 knots, the pilot monitoring pushed the throttles forward.

The blast from the engines spewed water up from the sea, but unlike internal combustion engines in motor vehicles, jet engines take time to spool up, and with the raised nose causing extra drag, the aircraft further slowed to 103 knots as it continued dropping. The control sticks then began shaking to warn of an imminent stall.

In the seven seconds remaining, the increasing thrust raised the airspeed by a mere three knots, not nearly enough to produce the lift required to fully arrest their descent let alone enable them to climb over the seawall, which the main landing gear struck violently, separating, as designed, from the aircraft without causing structural damage. The tip of the tail, even lower due to the nose-up attitude, struck the wall, too, with the tail cone shearing off along the line of the aft pressure bulkhead, just behind the four flight attendants sitting by the galley.

Because the aircraft had been just high enough for the landing gear to suffer and temper the initial impact, the aircraft hurtled on relatively intact for quite some distance before cartwheeling and coming to a stop with the wings still attached.

The gyrations subjected the fuselage to extreme lateral stresses, causing two evacuation slides on the right side to inflate inside the cabin without the hatches being opened. In doing so, they trapped the two flight attendants seated at those exits. One was about to suffocate when a member of the flight crew came with an axe from the cockpit to deflate the one trapping her, while a member of the cabin crew deflated the other with a knife from the galley.

Three Flight Attendants and 2 Passengers Ejected

Three of the four flight attendants sitting by the galley right at the rear just in front of the aft pressure bulkhead were ejected still strapped in their seats and survived, albeit seriously injured.

Two teenage girls sitting at the back whose seat belts were not attached were not so lucky on being ejected.

One, thrown out early on, probably died on impact with the ground, while the other, who was ejected just before the aircraft came to a stop, was twice run over by a fire appliance while lying covered by fire-retardant foam. There were two inquests, with the first finding she was still alive when run over, and the other not. This cast a shadow over the heroic efforts of the firefighters and notably those who climbed up the slides into the cabin to rescue five passengers unable to escape, one of whom later died.

The Evacuation

Ordering an evacuation is a decision not easily taken. Pilots sitting right at the front can see ahead but have little idea of what is going on behind them. Unless told by their instruments, they do not even know whether an engine is on fire.

In nose-up crash landings, where the tail suffers the initial impact, they can even believe it was a relatively smooth landing, when those right at the back are injured or killed. Most evacuations expose the occupants, and especially the older ones, to injury. Following protocol, the pilots liaised with the controllers in the tower, who had a clear view of the aircraft, and waited for communications from the cabin crew. Passengers were told to remain seated.

Though the engines had separated, one had ended up lying beside the fuselage by the right wing with its fuel tanks. Oil from a tank on it caught fire, and when the lead cabin attendant was informed of this, she ordered an evacuation—ninety seconds after the aircraft had come to a halt, ironically the time it should theoretically take for an airliner to be evacuated with only half the exits usable.

Only two out of four slides on the left deployed, but passengers were able to evacuate not only via them but also through the gap at the back where the tail cone had been. The lead flight attendant was praised by the rescuers for her professionalism and for having ensured everyone got out.

What with three cabin crew at the back having been ejected and others injured, only five were able to assist with the evacuation and help and, perhaps more importantly, control the passengers, some of whom, as they so often do, collected their luggage.

The fire finally penetrated the cabin, but firefighters who came in before it did much damage noted the seats at the front were pristine, while those right at the back were contorted.

Surprising Number of Survivors

On board there had been 12 crew and 291 passengers. Many of the passengers were Chinese, who had difficulty understanding what was happening. They included a group of teenagers on their way to a summer camp in the US who had the misfortune to be sitting at the back.

Surprisingly, 99 percent of the passengers survived, and only one passenger would have been killed—by a dislodged rear door—had all had their seat belts been attached. Altogether, 187 people were injured, of whom 49 were injured seriously. This is difficult to believe when one sees the videos taken from the control tower.

The Investigation

The NTSB's chair, Deborah Hersman, gave press conferences immediately after the event, leading to objections from ALPA (Air Line Pilots Association) that the release of information was leading to rampant speculation as to the cause.

Interestingly, she pointed out that exchanges between the pilots and the controllers are in the public domain, while material on the cockpit voice recorder is confidential and can only be made public as a transcript. In the author's view, this is a pity, as the tone of voice can reveal the atmosphere in the cockpit and the relationship between the pilots.

The accident happened essentially because the pilots failed to monitor the airspeed in the erroneous belief the autothrottle would ensure it was maintained at the target landing speed they had set.

However, this came about for a whole variety of reasons:

1. The pilots, in line with company policy, relied on automation whenever possible, and the pilot flying had never made a landing, even in visual conditions, without the help of the Autoland/ILS to keep him on the glide path. He was nervous, especially as he was being checked out and had performed less than perfectly on a previous check flight.

2. The Boeing documentation did not make it clear that the autothrottle did not control airspeed in "Hold" mode and that the clever safety feature whereby it would come to life in an emergency, such as a much-too-low airspeed, did not operate if one pilot's flight director was on and the other pilot's was off. The PF had previously flown Airbuses, which had different philosophies.

3. The check captain was performing that task for the first time and may not have had the confidence to order a go-around earlier.

4. Crew resource management was poor: the PF did not call out what he was doing. The pilot monitoring could perhaps have repeated his warning about the sink rate and should have concentrated on the instruments rather than, presumably, on the all-red PAPI lights outside.

Aftermath

The airline revised its training techniques to ensure pilots could better cope with flying manually. Boeing reviewed documentation and training so that the various autothrottle modes are better understood and followed NTSB advice to make low-airspeed warnings, for example, kick in earlier when the aircraft is near the ground and the time left to save the situation is limited.

Makers of escape slides strengthened their mechanisms to lessen the chance of them opening prematurely. Firefighters took measures to better manage accident zones and lessen the chance of injuring escaping passengers inadvertently.

Was Disappearance of MH370 Almost the Perfect Crime? (2014)

The greatest mystery since that of Amelia Earhart

> The Malaysian authorities' handling of the aftermath was so baffling that it is difficult to know whether it signified ineptitude or a cover-up.
>
> Malaysian Airlines Flight 370, March 8, 2014

MH370 was the Malaysian Airlines overnight flight from Kuala Lumpur to Beijing. The twelve-year-old Boeing 777 had a total of 53,460 hours but had been used on relatively long-haul routes and so only had 7,525 cycles, that is takeoffs and landings, which are what determines the age an aircraft in terms of metal fatigue. Bearing that in mind and that it had not been involved in an incident like a tail strike entailing major repairs, catastrophic failure of the fuselage was most unlikely.

Taking off from Kuala Lumpur's new airport at 00:41 Malaysia time with 12 crew and 267 passengers, it gradually gained height as it flew over the Malay Peninsula to the northeast.

At 01:06, just before reaching the coast, its ACARS data link automatically transmitted an update of its status, including the fact that 96,600 pounds (43,800 kilos) of fuel remained and that there were no faults. Out over the South China Sea, it reached its thirty-five-thousand-feet cruising height.

At 01:19, Kuala Lumpur air traffic control instructed them to switch frequency to that of the Vietnamese Ho Chi Minh air traffic control.

The captain of MH370 acknowledged and signed off by saying the haunting last words heard from the pilots:

Good night, Malaysian Three-Seven-Zero.

The Vietnamese controllers would not have been following their blip closely, as not having checked in there was nothing to say. Not having been listening in to the exchanges between MH370 and the Malaysian controllers they would not know exactly when to expect the call. Finally, when they thought it was taking far longer than expected, they could find no echo for MH370 on their screens.

Military radar, called primary radar, is designed to detect enemies from feeble waves reflected from the aircraft's surface. However, civilian air traffic control radar, called secondary radar, relies on a transponder on the aircraft to send back a much stronger echo with the identity, altitude, and airspeed of the aircraft. It also includes the four-figure squawk code assigned to the flight, which the pilot can change to, say, 7500 to report a hijacking, 7700 to indicate an emergency, or even 7600 for failure of the radio.

There was no blip for MH370 on the Vietnamese air traffic control radar. There was not even the ACARS data link.

ACARS (aircraft addressing and reporting system) is a data link that regularly sends information required for maintenance. Pilots can also use it for weather updates or even for requests, such as when medical assistance is needed for a disembarking passenger.

It can send the data cheaply via VHR radio or via satellite which is much more expensive, and for which Malaysian Airlines had not signed up. Even though Malaysian Airlines had not paid for satellite transmission, the satellite would at intervals "shake hands" with the onboard device so long as it had power.

It was not until 1:38, nineteen minutes after MH370 should have checked in, that Ho Chi Minh control called Kuala Lumpur ATC to ask what was happening, only to be informed MH370 had been told to contact them and signed off.

At 1:46, the Vietnamese again queried KL ATC, and were told there had been radar contact but no verbal contact at the IGARI waypoint. Ho Chi Minh replied that the radar blip had disappeared at BITOD, a waypoint slightly farther on.

At 1:50, KL ATC asked HCM ATC to confirm they had finally made contact and were told they had not. At 1:57, HCM informed KL ATC that they were declaring officially that there had never been any contact with MH370, despite direct calls on various frequencies and indirect attempts to contact them via other aircraft in the vicinity.

It was then that Malaysian Airlines Operations threw as spanner in the works by saying the aircraft was in Cambodian airspace, information that KL ATC duly passed on to HCM at 02:03.

Fifteen minutes later, at 02:18, a mystified KL controller asked HCM whether the flight plan happened to include a route through Cambodian airspace and was told it was solely through Vietnamese airspace, and that

HCM had checked with the Cambodians, only to be told they, too, had had no radar contact or communication with MH370.

At 3:30 Malaysia Airlines Operations staggeringly admitted that the coordinates they had given for MH370's location in Cambodia were merely based on projections and were not reliable for flight positioning, and KL duly informed HCM of this. At 4:25, HCM, obviously greatly concerned as MH370 should have passed through their patch, questioned KL as to whether they had heard anything from Hong Kong or Beijing!

At 4:30, KL ATC finally alerted search and rescue, which then, and for days, concentrated on the South China Sea off Vietnam and China, on the aircraft's scheduled route.

Where Had It Gone?

MH370, with the transponder not working or disabled, had in fact executed a U-turn and had long left the Vietnamese air traffic control area which it had in fact hardly entered. Thus, even search by primary radar would not have picked it up because they would be looking in the wrong place—in fact looking further along its route on the flight plan in the direction of Beijing.

Later analysis of Malaysian military radar showed it had flown back over the Malaysian Peninsula and not to Kuala Lumpur but to Penang, farther north, then turned right to fly northwest up the Strait of Malacca beyond the tip of Sumatra where there was no military radar coverage either from Malaysia or Indonesia.

Inmarsat

Several days later, experts from the satellite telecommunications company Inmarsat were able to show it must have turned left just beyond the tip of Sumatra and flown in a southerly direction, to come down hours later somewhere in the southern Indian Ocean perhaps two thousand miles off Perth, Australia.

Even when it became known the aircraft had not crashed in the South China Sea the Malaysian authorities persisted with the search there not only wasting the time and money of countries deploying their aircraft and ships but delaying the search in more likely places.

What Had Happened?

The briefings by the Malaysian authorities were a disaster, perhaps partly because knowing little and understanding less they gave premature answers to incredulous Chinese relatives. Usually when there is a crash, people know where it was and roughly what happened, giving relatives something to latch onto and allowing them to accept the assertion, justified or not, that the investigators cannot say much. Here there was nothing to investigate.

The Malaysian military were accused of being slack, though again, to be fair, one must admit that relatively junior officers would understandably hesitate to send up fighters to investigate nonthreatening blips in the middle of the night without their superiors' authorization, and particularly so if the blip was exiting the country and obviously not a threat.

Reports their radar operators had seen the aircraft climbing to a great height—supposedly to incapacitate the passengers—and descending and climbing steeply were later discounted, since doing so would have used so much fuel that that the 777 could not have flown for as long as it did.

Also, it was alleged the military in neighboring countries were keeping quiet so as not to divulge what they could see, or as others said, more likely not to reveal how little they could see.

The Captain
The captain was fifty-three-year-old Zaharie Ahmad Shah from Penang. The fact that the aircraft flew over Penang on its way out to the Indian Ocean led to suggestions that he was committing suicide and wanted a last look at the place where he had been brought up. Penang also had a long runway that would have made it a good place to head for to make an emergency landing.

Zaharie had 18,365 flying hours on various aircraft, including many on the 777. He loved flying and had a flight simulator at home. However, one must be wary of taking comments by family members at face value, as it is in their interest, even financial, to show their relative must be innocent.

An insight into Zaharie's character may be gained from reports in September 2018 said analysis of his social media activities revealed the mental status of a man psychologists say was "self-destructive." During 2013, the fifty-three-year-old made ninety-seven separate Facebook comments directed at twenty-six-year-old twin sisters Lan Qi Hui and Qi Min Lan (who had hundreds of thousands of followers just on Instagram) were largely ignored. Zaharie implored the twins to come to Kuala Lumpur, where he lived with his wife. "When in KL," he wrote, "How about KL." In one he suggestively said, "Just showered?"

Zaharie's behavior was somewhat over the top, even timewise. Could it mean there might be other cases that could prove embarrassing or even impact him professionally, as happened to the Egyptian pilot who committed suicide? But was it really "self-destructive" behavior, as claimed by the psychologists cited by the media?

The Copilot
The copilot was twenty-seven-year-old Fariq Ab Hamid, from Kuala Lumpur. Though it was only his sixth flight in the 777 and the first time without being supervised by a check pilot, he had 2,763 flying hours, having joined the airline in 2007.

Nothing suggested he was a man going to commit suicide. He was about to wed his wonderful fiancée, a captain flying for the low-cost airline AirAsia, whom he had known ever since they had been students at Langkawi Flying School. He was a relaxed fun-loving type if one is to believe the photos given to the media by two South African teenage girls showing them sitting with him in the cockpit and them all laughing and smoking away.

Military Radar—Track Back over the Malaysian Peninsula

Although it was not known or revealed until later, the Malaysian military had seen the aircraft, as mentioned, turn left after passing the IGARI waypoint, which is near a point where three air traffic control regions—those of Malaysia, Vietnam, and Singapore—meet, so that the aircraft is in a zone where it is effectively under the control of the center actually handling it. Also, VHF radio, used both for voice and ACARS communications, can be intermittent, which may in part make controllers wait for communications to improve before worrying or ask other aircraft to make contact for them.

It had flown back over the Malaysian Peninsula, over Penang, before turning almost forty-five degrees to the right to go up the Strait of Malacca without passing over land. It then went out of Malaysian military radar range.

Satellite Handshakes

Malaysian Airlines had not paid for ACARS data to be transmitted via satellite, but the satellites nevertheless performed handshakes at regular intervals to confirm the system was working should it be required, whereby the satellite transmits a signal (a ping) and waits for a reply (a pong).

Following the disappearance of Air France flight AF447 over the South Atlantic, where the company was paying for satellite transmission of ACARS data, Inmarsat, the British company providing the service, found there was not enough information about the aircraft's location and incorporated a timing feature in the handshake that could give some general indication of the location.

This new feature provided the startling news that MH370 had flown on for almost six hours after being lost from view on radar near the northern tip of Indonesia. The satellite, hovering at thirty-five thousand kilometers above the ocean, showed the aircraft must have come down on one of two arcs, one to the north, the other to the south. The northern one was discounted because wide-ranging military radar coverage there was such that it could never have been missed for so long.

The conclusion was that it had come down off Perth, Australia, in an isolated area with terrible sea conditions known as the Roaring Forties.

Much time had been lost looking in the South China Sea, and the locator beacons, which only last thirty days, were almost out of power when the proper search began. There were moments when it was thought signals had been picked up, but these proved to be red herrings.

Aircraft from various nations scoured the surface of the sea for debris without finding any that could ultimately be proved to be from the aircraft. Had the search concentrated on that area earlier, there would of course have been a better chance of finding something. Recently, some French satellite images have appeared showing items in the water that could be man-made, but definition was too poor to draw definitive conclusions as to what they might be.

Debris—Flaperon with Trailing Edge Broken Off
On July 29, 2015, sixteen months after MH370's disappearance, a flaperon from the aircraft was found on a beach in Saint-André, on Réunion, off Madagascar.

Reference numbers made its origin virtually certain and dashed the hopes of relatives that their loved ones might be still alive.

The trailing edge of the flaperon had clearly broken off, something requiring considerable force, making some conclude the flaps had been deployed by a human so the aircraft would come down relatively gently under control and not break up into thousands of pieces. Indeed, a part of a flap was later found in the same general area with the trailing edge similarly broken off.

A small amount of other debris was found, all of which could have been brought there by currents from where the aircraft supposedly went down.

The flaperon was sent to France, and the French were keeping it on the grounds that it is evidence in a judicial inquiry and that La Réunion is French territory.

The Underwater Searches

The location of the presumed final resting place meant that Malaysia, with its limited resources, was in charge of the investigation, and though an expensive underwater search, managed by Australia, was undertaken with vessels and equipment mainly from China and Australia, Malaysia was obviously a partner. After two years' searching in extremely difficult conditions, it was called off, just as revised wreckage-drift analysis and rethinks regarding the satellite data and the possible point where the turn to the south Indian Ocean was made suggest more certainty as to the likely resting place of sunk wreckage from the flight on the ocean floor.

Hopes were high when on January 10, 2018, Malaysia's government announced it would pay Texas-based Ocean Infinity up to $70 million if it could find the wreckage or black boxes of Malaysia Airlines Flight 370 within three months. Unfortunately, despite the deployment of eight underwater drones able to stay under water for forty-eight hours at a time—which unlike those used in previous searches are not tethered to the surface ship by cable and reduce noise to yield data of better quality—the search was unsuccessful.

For the relatives, finding the aircraft and their loved ones, and hopefully determining who might be responsible for such a dastardly thing, is of prime importance.

For others, and from an air safety point of view, it may be less so, as the aircraft flew on for hours with changes of course unlike Air France Flight 447 lost in the South Atlantic after dropping out of the sky while still on course and with the ACARS link working. There were fears and accusations at the time that there was something inherently wrong with the Airbus A330, making it of the utmost interest for the manufacturer and the French government to prove otherwise. In the end, discovery of the wreckage and recovery of the recorders after two years proved the pilots had turned a glitch into a disaster.

Even recovering MH370's cockpit voice recorder would not reveal how the incident was orchestrated, for to protect pilot privacy, CVRs overwrite themselves at half- or in this case two-hour intervals. Passengers' mobile phones might provide answers, but not if they died through lack of oxygen before there was anything of note to see.

Searching for the Truth

Analyzing the satellite data regarding the location of descent into the sea and associated evidence is extremely complex, and a subject for specialists.

Though interpretation of the satellite data gives some idea of along what arc MH370 came down, that is a line thousands of miles long. Where on that line, and how far away from it to search, was based on how far the aircraft could go with the fuel it had and whether someone might have flown it away from that line after the fuel ran out. Complicating the issue is the fact that after going northwest up the Strait of Malacca, MH370 may have continued much farther than thought before turning south. An extra fifteen minutes would mean almost half an hour's difference in flying time to the south, meaning the expensive underwater search had been much too far south.

Also, if the pilot had recovered the aircraft after it had dived after running out of fuel, he (or even she) could have glided a fair distance to either side of the arc, making the search area much vaster. More recent drift analysis based on the few pieces of wreckage found suggest the aircraft had come down further north on the arc than previously assumed.

Anyone fascinated and wanting to keep up to date technically might well visit Victor Iannello's *http://mh370.radiantphysics.com/* website. An American engineer living in Virginia, Iannello has been passionately following the affair. His blogs are not for the faint-hearted and much too technical for most, but some of the comments on them make fascinating points, besides revealing how many different points of view there are, with people getting quite worked up, and even angry.

Interestingly, data released almost three years after the event to one of the next of kin contained all of the information transmitted via an Inmarsat satellite link on the previous flight by the jet, from Beijing to Kuala Lumpur, picking up features that were common to both flights and not anomalies unique to MH370.

Tentative Conclusion (Summary)

Taken individually, many of the twists and turns are explicable, but taken as a whole, the coincidences, leading to suspicion it was an intentional act, are just too many:

1. It all started seemingly all too conveniently just after 01:19 Malaysia time at the point where the Malaysian and Vietnamese flight information regions (FIRs) intersect. Having just left Malaysian control, MH370 disappeared from civilian radar without having signed on with the Vietnamese. Not only had the transponder stopped working, the ACARS data link had, too. Though they could have reversed course to get back to Malaysia to make an emergency landing, it also meant the Vietnamese controllers would be looking for them, possibly with primary military radar, in quite the wrong place.

2. Because they turned left some 150 degrees to
    Penang, rather than 180 degrees back to Kuala
    Lumpur, the possibility of the unidentified aircraft
    being suspected as having been hijacked and about
    to be flown into the Petronas twin towers, 9/11-
    style, was avoided.
3. Turning to the right after Penang to go north up
    the Strait of Malacca avoided drawing the attention
    of the Indonesians.
4. Malaysian radar tracked them going up the strait
    until 02:22, after which they turned left on reaching
    some point above the northern tip of Sumatra, to fly
    south over the ocean to one of the most remote
    parts of the world, where, without the satellite
    handshake data, no one would ever dream of
    looking. Last satellite contact was at 08:19, seven
    hours after "Goodnight, Malaysian Three-Seven-
    Zero."

Was someone trying to prove how clever they were by
creating what Victor Iannello's blog calls "the world's
greatest aviation mystery"? If one rules out the about-to-
be-married first officer, who had shown a love for the
good things in life, that only leaves the technically minded
captain, unless there was a rogue passenger or someone
hiding on board, even in the avionics bay. If he was
genius-like going to create the greatest-ever aviation
mystery he surely would be clever enough to hide his
anger from his spouse.

Since the cockpit voice recorder records on a two-hour loop, if it is recovered it will probably only reveal whether someone was breathing, praying, or ranting at the very end. On the other hand, that person, at the very least, might be identifiable.

Final Australian Report

On October 3, 2017, the Australian National Transport Safety Bureau (ATSB) issued its lengthy final report on MH370, or rather, on its role relating to the unsuccessful 1,046-day underwater search off Australia. We were lucky to be able to use the information in the report in writing this piece.

It was not the FBI, as rumored, but a Malaysian contractor that the Malaysian authorities engaged as part of a police investigation, the details of which were never made public, that analyzed the captain's home computer and found traces of a simulated maneuver far south in the Indian Ocean.

An Emirates airliner going northwest up the Strait of Malacca just thirty-three nautical miles behind MH370 had the same track on the military radar, confirming the latter was also following the waypoints like a normal flight.

If the intention was to commit suicide creating the greatest mystery in aviation, one must wonder how someone reasonably clever could do it at the expense of so many.

Final Malaysian Report (July 30, 2018)

The 400-page final official Malaysian report revealed little of note other than that the initial 180-degree turn was made manually because the autopilot could not have done that in 2 minutes 10 seconds and that the transponder stopped transmitting, "whether with intent or otherwise." Adding "Although it cannot be conclusively ruled out that an aircraft or system malfunction was a cause, based on the limited evidence available, it is more likely that the loss of communication prior to the diversion is due to the systems being manually turned off or power interrupted to them."

It virtually dismissed the idea that the pilots could be responsible, saying that there was no sign of stress in their radio communications and investigators had found no evidence of anything suspicious regarding them. However, someone able to do something "so clever" could be clever enough to conceal their state of mind. There have been cases where—without proof—investigators have concluded an accident has been caused by far the most likely cause only to be later proved totally wrong. In this case we must be wary of assuming the most likely scenario based on indirect evidence is necessarily what happened.

August 2018—Reaction to the Report
In response to the final official report by the Malaysian investigators on July 30, 2018, the research section of the French Air Transport Police announced it would conduct its own review of the satellite data (pings from the aircraft) as there had been four French citizens on board, and verifying it was necessary for their investigation. This implied they were not satisfied.

Publication of the report was also an occasion for the world's media to regurgitate the many theories regarding what might have happened, including the suggestion a stowaway might have been hiding in the avionics bay (accessible from the ground and via a hatch behind the cockpit), and the possibility that the aircraft could have been taken over electronically by hackers. About the latter, Boeing said that although it had patented a remote-control system as a possible way to take control away from hijackers such as those in 9/11, it had not installed such a system on any commercial aircraft.

The Malaysian report said the first officer's mobile phone had been on and had made a handshake at Penang with no call, and that tests had been made showing that was possible. Some experts were surprised no attempts were made to see whether any of the Malaysian passengers' phones had similarly tried to log on to a Malaysian mobile phone network, as at least one or two passengers tend to leave their phones on.

It also noted "no traces of explosion were found" on two pieces of debris that almost certainly came from the cabin interior.

Malaysia's civil aviation chief resigned after the report, which found failures by Malaysian air traffic control, notably lapses by controllers in relation to emergency procedures. The aircraft had been missing, the report said, for about twenty minutes before authorities sent an alert. As he was close to retirement anyway, his resignation was not so meaningful.

The mystery is as great, if not greater, than ever.

In some ways it resembles the mystery of the disappearance of Amelia Earhart, with which we began this book, in that those hooked on the case regularly come up with reasoned but mostly wild theories and "finds" that are given full-blown coverage in the media with headlines suggesting that the truth or wreckage may at last have been found.

Part 3 of this large print edition will have updates but whether these will include mention of the discovery of the wreckage of MH370 is questionable.

Index

Updates including recent accidents

will be placed in

PART 3
Glossary & Flying Dictionary

for which there will also be a Kindle Version

How to Purchase

To find the appropriate version on Amazon go to our website *https://chrisbart.com* and click on the appropriated link next to the Table of Contents."

Also available from bookshops but usually must be specially ordered.

Online Shop for Multiple Copies

Flying schools, associations, clubs, and individuals wishing to buy a several copies for training or as presents, may find it very advantageous to purchase from the shop on our website *https://chrisbart.com*. Unfortunately, we can only arrange for deliveries in the countries where the books are printed, namely Australia, the UK, and the US (Mainland).

www.ingramcontent.com/pod-product-compliance
Lightning Source LLC
Chambersburg PA
CBHW031939080426
42735CB00007B/192